# THE BOOK OF JOANN
A Novel Based on Her Life Story, and the Lifetime Battle She Endured with Mental Illness

## LISA ZARCONE

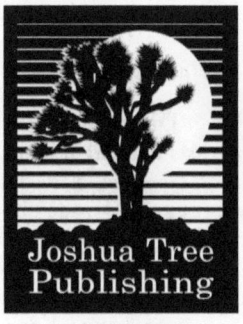

• Chicago •

# THE BOOK OF JOANN
## A Novel Based on Her Life Story, and the Lifetime Battle She Endured with Mental Illness
### LISA ZARCONE

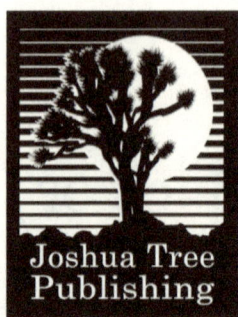

Published by
**Joshua Tree Publishing**
• Chicago •
JoshuaTreePublishing.com

All rights reserved. No part of this book may be reproduced or transmitted in any form or by any means, electronic or mechanical, including information storage and retrieval system without written permission from the publisher, except by a reviewer who may quote brief passages in a review.

13-Digit Print ISBN: 978-1-956823-53-0
Copyright © 2024 Lisa Zarcone. All Rights Reserved.
Front Cover Credits:   New Africa Adobe Stock (daffodils)
                                       photohampster Adobe Stock (Clover))

**Disclaimer:**
This book is designed to provide information about the subject matter covered. The opinions and information expressed in this book are those of the author, not the publisher. Every effort has been made to make this book as complete and as accurate as possible. However, there may be mistakes both typographical and in content. Therefore, this text should be used only as a general guide and not as the ultimate source of information. The author and publisher of this book shall have neither liability nor responsibility to any person or entity with respect to any loss or damage caused or alleged to be caused directly or indirectly by the information contained in this book.

Printed in the United States of America

# Dedication

I want to dedicate this story to my mother Joann Sega. Her life was an unbelievable experience unless you walked that road with her to witness it for yourself. She was a tenacious woman with high intelligence and a bold personality. As a woman with deep faith, she loved her family fiercely.

I would not have been able to write this story without her willingness to share each and every experience of her life, long before me. Her story is a true testament of strength, faith, courage, and the ability to laugh at the darkness she faced daily.

I am so proud of this book, and my accomplishment to fulfill the promise that I made to her so many years ago. She wanted her story to be shared, so people would truly understand what mental illness looks like from all angles of life. I know she is proud of me, and her legacy will always live on through every word on these pages.

I love you mom, and I am grateful to have had the gift of seeing you for who you truly were. You were a woman who just wanted to be a loving mother and experience the goodness that life had to offer. It is unfortunate that mental illness robbed us both of those positive experiences.

I treasure every wonderful moment and the great conversations we had along the way.

I am proud to be your daughter.

\* \* \*

To my husband John, the love of my life and my soul mate. I want to thank you so very much for walking this path with me. You have supported me in every way a husband should, and so much more. You always believed in me, even when I didn't believe in myself—and for that I am forever grateful.

You showed my mother love and compassion, even on her worst days. As you stood by my side painfully watching me suffer from the backlash of Joann, you also continued to try to understand her pain as well. You are a remarkable man, and I know God sent you my way for a reason.

Please know that I love you more than words could ever say, and I feel so blessed to have you by my side always. You are an amazing gift!

Thank you all who continue to show up for me as we walk forward together.

This story is always dedicated to all who suffer with mental health struggles, and I hope by reading Joann's story, you know that you are not alone.

Please reach out for help and support when you need it, and remember it is OK to say the words out loud. You are worthy of great things in life.

Embrace the Journey.
God Bless

Lisa Rose (Sega) Zarcone

# Acknowledgements

Lisa Zarcone, author of "The Unspoken Truth," and I connected months after I broke my silence and went public about my history of surviving childhood sexual abuse. I reached out to her several years ago, after hearing about her book and her tireless advocacy on behalf of warriors fighting to reclaim their lives. Her next book, " The Book of Joann," is an honest, powerful read about the impact of having a mother who struggled with mental illness. Lisa promised her mother that she would share her story to help the world gain deeper understanding of mental illness and its profound impact on others. I continue to be inspired by Lisa's bravery and determination and how she uses her experience of surviving childhood trauma to help so many others.

**Shari Botwin**, LCSW, author of *Thriving After Trauma* and upcoming book, *Stolen Childhoods*. (www.sharibotwin.com)

~

Lisa Zarcone is a true advocate of Mental Health for all. She stops at nothing to help people avoid struggling with mental health or helping those who are currently struggling to navigate through their tough times. Whether it's a motivational post on social media or one of her awesome written articles, Lisa has a story that needs to be told and heard by others. She is a special person who has been chosen to make change in the world to help people with their Mental Health journey. Lisa and I met on social media and travel down the same path. We always hope that our voices and messages are heard by all.

**Eric Daddario** — Youth Mental Health advocate Speaker

~

Lisa Zarcone is a remarkable, courageous woman, mental health and child abuse advocate whom I've had the pleasure of getting to know, respect and admire. She was a featured guest on my Power Your Life Radio Show revealing her personal experiences with her mother's mental health illness and its impact on her as a child in The Unspoken Truth memoir. Despite how difficult it was to share her experiences, Lisa wanted to bring awareness to mental health challenges and protect the safety of others, especially children. It's no accident that our paths have crossed. I have been an advocate for children and youth with special needs, anti-bullying and neurodiversity to bring more acceptance, understanding and inclusion for people stigmatized by their differences. Our connection over time has deepened. I am excited that Lisa's new book "The Book of Joann" is based on a promise given to her mother: To disclose her mother's story of mental illness and how it affected her life and that of Lisa, her child. Through authentic stories, people can see firsthand the debilitating effects of mental illness, gain awareness and support mental health and child abuse safety. We can only shift and shape what we know. For too long, mental illness and child abuse were kept hidden. Now is the time to awaken people so real change can take place.

**Dr. Jo Anne White**, International #1 bestselling, award winning author, speaker, consultant and Goodwill Global Ambassador for civil and humanitarian work in education, entrepreneurship, coaching and women's issues, life, spiritual, leadership and business coach and Executive Producer and Host of the POWER YOUR LIFE Shows.

~

Lisa Zarcone and I met in 2018 after publishing our first books and we connected immediately. Whilst our books had different stories, they shared a common theme: living a life shattered by child abuse, mental illness and suicidal ideation. Since our first meeting, Lisa and I have worked tirelessly sharing our stories and creating awareness about mental illness/health and child abuse/safety. I am so proud of Lisa, despite all that is happening in her life and in the world, she has never stopped her advocacy work; never waivered in her vision to be a voice for children and adults, to educate children and adults, and to listen to and help anyone impacted by child abuse, mental illness, suicide. I am excited to read her new book, The Book of Joann!

I know this story will be powerful, heartbreaking, and insightful. Kudos Lisa, for sharing your mother's story and creating awareness about living with mental illness.

**Tracey Maxfield**
Retired Nurse, Mental Health/Stop Bullying Advocate, Author
*Escaping the Rabbit Hole: My Journey Through Depression*

To my dear friend and mentor Lisa Zarcone, the one who found me many years ago advocating for my son's mental health and convinced me to share my story on a podcast. You are an incredible woman filled with courage, strength, resilience and a true inspiration to me and so many others out there.

A quote from my book that I believe applies so much to you as well,

"For every pain, there is wisdom; for every loss, there is gain, and for every tear, there is purpose. I, determined to write this book and use my experience, wisdom, research, and resultant strength to be a force for change."

Lisa, your first book was incredible, to have to dig deep into your past and relive such horrifying abuse, well only a very strong person can do something like that. To be able to forgive the main source of your abuse, your mother, and then to write about her in your newest book, that is resilience. I'm honored to be your friend and fellow Author.

XOXO Always

**Bailey Smith** @marriedtoanillusion

~

Lisa Zarcone is a lady who has been through the refiner's fire. Having survived childhood sexual, verbal, and mental abuse, she has shown amazing resilience in rising above tremendous adversity. Rather than letting that adversity crush her, she has used it as a steppingstone to stand up, speak out, and ignite awareness about what it takes to thrive as an adult who survived childhood abuse. Lisa and I connected a few years ago when we interviewed her for The Kindness & Happiness Connection podcast. It was her courage to speak out that inspired me to have the courage to share my own survival story. It's the Lisa Zarcone's of the world that make it a better place to live in!

**Randy McNeely**, author of *The Kindness Givers' Formula 2.0: A 5-Step Guide for Reaching Hearts, Inspiring Change, and Healing the World Through Love*

# Table of Contents

| | |
|---|---:|
| Dedication | 3 |
| Acknowledgements | 5 |
| A Walk Back in Time | 11 |
| The Teenage Years—Challenging Times | 22 |
| Here Comes the Children | 31 |
| Time Marches On | 41 |
| The Breakdown | 48 |
| Time in the Psychiatric Unit—Hell On Earth | 53 |
| Middle Town Psychiatric Unit | 59 |
| Transition Back To The Real World | 67 |
| Fall Is Upon Us—The Great Depression | 77 |
| When Leukemia Strikes | 84 |
| The Stories of My Youth | 100 |
| The Battle Of The Wills—Mother vs Daughter | 127 |
| The Fury Raged On | 134 |
| Catch Me If You Can | 141 |
| Transitions | 147 |
| Growing Up In Spite of Joann | 153 |
| Not A Child Anymore—Time in a bottle . . . | 161 |
| A Battle For Freedom | 166 |
| The Next Stage of Life | 174 |
| The Cracks | 179 |
| Off To The Nursing Home—The Next Stage Of Life | 195 |
| The Damaged Relationship | 204 |
| The Time Is Now | 212 |
| Epilogue—"24" | 218 |
| About the Author | 222 |

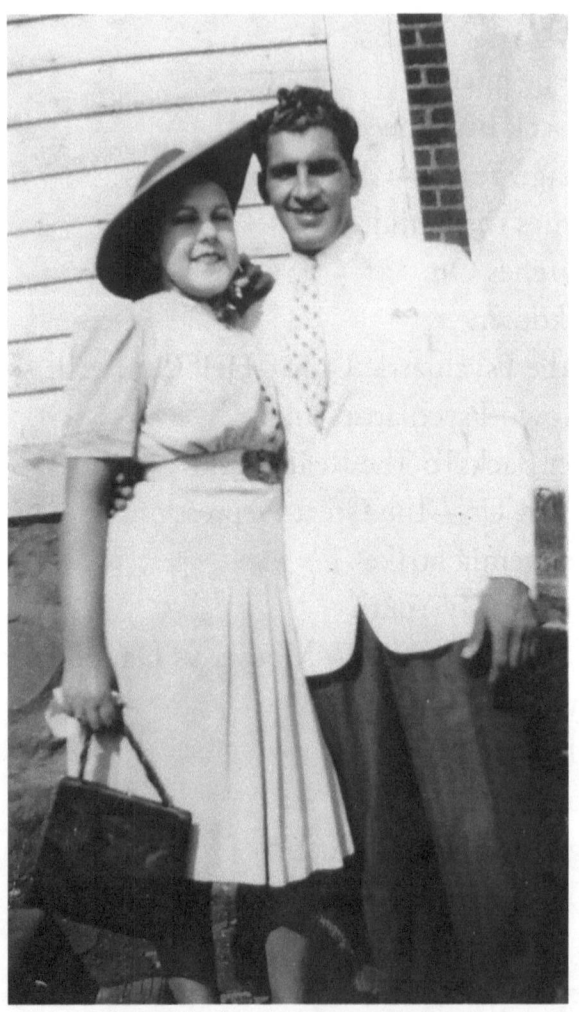

*Joann's Parents Rose and Pat*

# Chapter 1

# A Walk Back in Time

Joann Helen, my mother, was born on June 24, 1941, on a sunny day in New Haven, Connecticut. She would be the oldest of four children. She was a beautiful young girl with light brown ringlets in her hair and chocolate-brown eyes almond shaped to perfection. She was slender in shape and loved to dress pretty.

As my mother made her way forward throughout her childhood, the early signs of mental illness were there, but during that era, it was not something that was talked about—or even acknowledged. As a child, my mother struggled tremendously with anxiety, fear, and mood swings.

When all the other children were outside playing, including her younger sister, most of the time you would find Joann sitting in the upstairs window of this six-family home, picking at the chipped paint and talking to her cat, Chooch. She would sit with her grandmother, who was blind, keeping her company and helping to take care of her. Instead of being a happy go lucky child running and playing throughout the neighborhood, there she sat with her anxiety and sadness quietly building. Watching all the other children laughing and playing was very hard for her to endure because she knew she could not participate because of duty and her own debilitating mind.

Imagine at eight years old knowing you are different; feeling it but not being able to express it. Little Joann found comfort in taking care of her grandmother. She loved to listen to her grandmother talk and sing in Italian. This was the creative reason that she gave to the neighborhood children as an excuse not to come outside and play. She came up with this idea so they would not pick on her—or see her true disabilities. At week's end, she was paid a nickel for her work, and she happily put it in her jar. As she collected her money, she would sometimes make her way to the corner store to buy penny candy for her and her sister.

Happily, she would skip down the street, feeling a moment of peace and freedom, as she smiled thinking about what she would be able to buy with her earnings. This was a routine that she became comfortable with, and she felt a little bit stronger doing something on her own. Joann's confidence was slowly building, but that soon would be shattered by circumstance.

On this one hot summer day, she announced to her mother that she was going to run down to the store to get her candy, and she would return soon. As her mom happily sent her on her way, she told her, "Joann be careful and watch out when you cross the street!"

"I will, mommy," was her response.

As the hot sun beat down on her face, her nose crinkled as she hated to be hot or sweaty. You see, Joann was a girly girl who enjoyed wearing pretty little dresses with her hair just so. The thought of being sweaty bothered her tremendously, but she put those feelings aside as she listened to the birds chirping, the children's laughter, and the hustle and bustle of cars passing by. The aroma of freshly baked bread filled the air as she made her way to the corner store. Joann smiled brightly, as she loved the smell of homemade Italian bread. It even made her little tummy do a grumbling dance. She touched her tummy and giggled.

As she made her way into the store, she took a long sniff of that fabulous bread as it was just pulled out of the oven. Then her thoughts shifted to the mission at hand, and her excitement grew at the thought of buying some Laffey Taffy and Root Beer barrels.

She marched her way directly to the candy section, as the old man behind the counter greeted her with a sheepish smile.

"Oh, I see you are here for your weekly candy."

Little Joann nodded shyly, barely giving him eye contact, feeling his eyes upon her, as she began to feel a bit uncomfortable.

"What a pretty little girl you are, and I love your dress."

Without a response, she nodded again, picking out her candy, now feeling a bit panicked, as this man never spoke a word to her in the countless times she had shopped at the store.

He then made his way around to the front of the counter to get a bit closer to her, and she completely froze.

"I have something special that I would like to show you. Would you like to see it?"

"No, I just want to buy my candy and go home now please," Joann quietly muttered.

He then grabbed her by the arm and said, "Shhh" as he aggressively pulled her into the back room, exposing his penis, then forcing her to touch it.

In sheer terror, she tried to scream but not a sound came out, as she was riddled with total fear. Once she was finally able to get the words out of her mouth, she let out a blood curdling scream, "Stop it! Stop it! Let me go!"

She startled him enough that he did let her go because he also heard the bell ring as a customer was coming in the front door. That was when she took her moment and ran as fast as she could out of that creepy back room, passing the in-coming customer, completely dropping her candy everywhere.

Then, like a flash, out the door she flew with tears in her eyes, as she ran all the way home. When she hit the steps of her big brown apartment complex, she began to hyperventilate, dropping down to the wooden steps, as her little legs could not carry her another step. The sheer terror in her eyes would have told anyone that she was in danger.

After a few moments, she was able to compose herself enough to get up and make her way upstairs to the comfort of her home and her mother. As she burst through the door, her little heart was beating out of her chest. The slamming of the door startled her mother, and she jumped up.

"Joann, what is wrong, and where is your candy?"

Joann burst into tears, crying so hard that she could not even speak. Her mother was not too alarmed at first, as her daughter could be a huge drama queen, but she quickly realized that this was quite a bit different. Joann was now in a complete panic attack, barely able to breathe.

Her mother was a very strong woman who did not get spooked very easily. Rose was a charismatic Italian woman filled with intelligence and common sense. She would rationalize everything. She stood about five-feet-four, a little stocky. She was starting to go blind like her own mother, but that did not stop her tenacity, spunk, and fiery spirit. Rose was a dark-haired beauty with a round face and button nose. She was stern at times but displayed her nurturing qualities when needed. On this day, she comforted her daughter and asked her to tell her what happened.

Once Joann was finally calm enough to share her story, it was one that her mother was not expecting to hear at all!

She was furious, but not at her daughter. It was pure rage and anger directed at the perverted, old fool at the corner store.

Rose took her daughter next door to her mother's apartment and said to her, "Stay here, I will take care of this matter immediately!"

Joann ran to the window to watch her mother march down the street towards the corner store. With fear in her eyes, she began to shake as the sweat trickled down her body. Her grandmother asked her what was going on in Italian. She did not speak English very well, but Joann understood her fully and explained briefly what happened. Her grandmother sighed but did not say a word.

Rose marched right into that store and confronted the store owner, who adamantly denied the accusations. Rose went on to say, "If you ever touch my daughter again, there will be hell to pay!"

With fire in her eyes, he knew she meant business. She went on to say that they would never step foot in his store again, and he lost all of their business, as other customers looked on in disbelief.

Rose did not care what other people were thinking. This was her child, and she was a fierce lion in that moment protecting her cub. Of course, during this time frame, the late '40s, it was not proper for a woman to speak in such a tone, especially to a man, but in that moment, nobody was going to question her virtue. When she was done reprimanding the old pig, she turned around and marched right back out of the store slamming the door with great force.

From the window, Joann saw her mom coming back, and some relief began to wash over her, as she shouted out loud, "Here comes mommy!"

"Good," her grandmother bellowed in Italian. "I am sure she took care of it!"

Rose made her way upstairs, collected her daughter, and went back into the apartment.

"Don't worry Joann. That man will never bother you again, and you are not allowed to ever go back to that store. Do you hear me?"

"Yes mommy, I am sorry."

Her mother walked back into the kitchen to cook dinner, and it was never talked about again. Joann never received an explanation as to why this old man would do such a thing to her, and she felt for some reason it was all her fault.

When she apologized to her mother for what happened, her mom never said to her, "Don't worry. It was not your fault. It was his."

Joann felt deep-seated guilt over this altercation. Unfortunately, this was a theme that carried on inside of her throughout her whole life.

This was the beginning of when little Joann began to struggle on new levels, and the ugly head of mental illness would begin to pop out, without warning. There were anger, self-doubt, mean-spirited actions and tears, many misunderstood tears.

As a young girl, she was confused by what had happened, and there was no opportunity to share her anger, fear, or guilt. Again, the sign of the times!

Unfortunately, this was not the only time that Joann was exposed to inappropriate behavior by an older man. Sadly, to say, the next event hit much closer to home.

\* \* \*

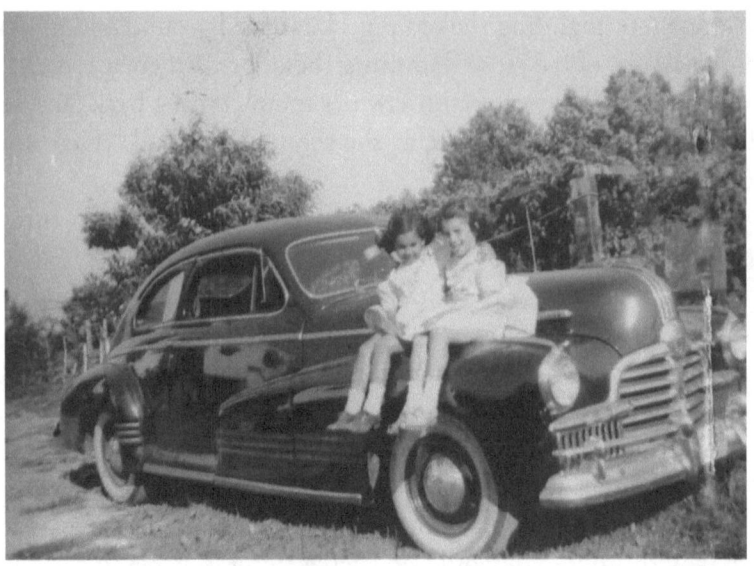

*Up the Country Road Joann*

Joann's father came from a big family of farmers, and on Sundays, the family would all gather at the farm, up on the hill in West Haven. They owned several acres of land which they used for a variety of things. They had huge gardens, rows of apple and pear trees, a beautiful grape arbor, and a huge red barn for the animals. As the family would gather to eat, drink, and play music, the kids would run amuck all over the property, picking blackberries, raspberries, and blue berries. Their little stained fingers and brightly colored tongues were proof of their full bellies!

One day when the kids were playing hide and seek, Joann went into the barn to hide among the cows, and she ran directly into her grandfather. He was an older Italian man with very chiseled features, dark skin, and bushy red hair. He was not a kind man and always had a stern look of disgust on his face. He grumbled under his breath with such anger when she bumped into him.

"Sorry, Grandpa. I didn't see you standing there. We are playing hide and seek."

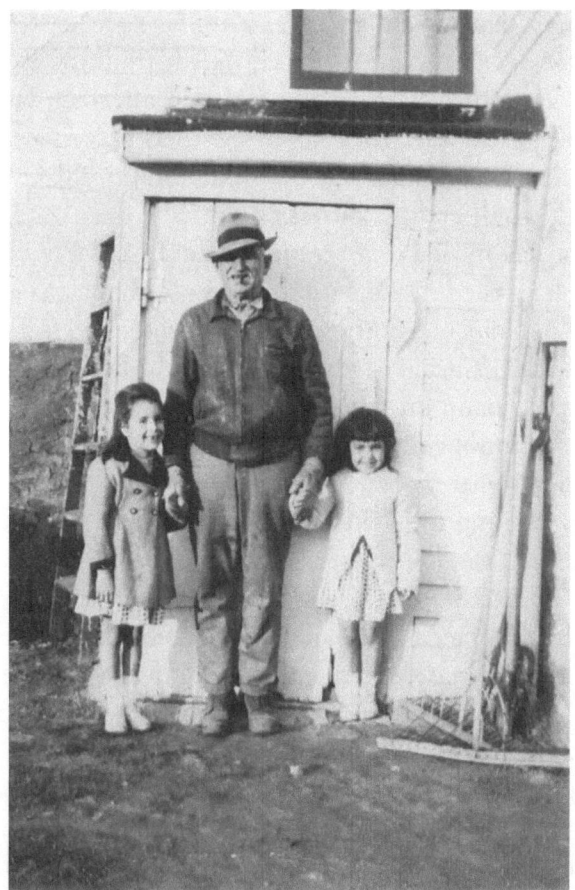

*Joann, Grandfather, and Cousin*

He mumbled something in Italian as his eyes grew big and scary. Then he grabbed her, swooping her up in his arms, squeezing her very tightly as he carried her to the back side of the barn. He dropped her with such force that she bounced when she hit the ground covered in hay.

She was frightened by his strength and brute force as he squeezed her so tightly. He smelled of dirty sweat and cow manure, which turned her stomach. Now acknowledging the pain from her fall and feeling a bit stunned, she was looking up at him with fear in her eyes as he abruptly dropped his pants, ready to make a move on her, but he was interrupted when the cousins began calling out to her as they were making their way into the barn. Joann quickly jumped to her feet and high tailed it out of there running right past her cousins. They looked at her confused but chuckled, thinking it was part of the game. They turned around and chased after her, laughing and giggling the whole way. They never saw their perverted grandfather standing there with his pants at his ankles, frantically grasping so he could quickly pull up his trousers!

As the day moved forward, Joann never said a word to anyone as to what happened in the barn, but she could not wait to go home. She would not look at her grandfather, but she could feel him staring at her. She felt his burning glare screaming at her without him ever saying a word. Joann knew she must remain silent or else.

"Please can we go home now. I do not feel good, my stomach is sick," she said to her mom.

After whining for a little bit, her mom said, "Gather up your sister, and I will get your father, move quickly"

That is exactly what Joann did, and soon they were making their way back home, as her parents were completely annoyed by her behavior. The car was dead silent. You could cut the tension with a knife. Joann looked over at her sister who glared at her because she did not want to leave—she was having fun.

When the car pulled into the driveway, Joann was the first one out making her way up the stairs, running to the safety of her apartment and cat. It was like a repeat scenario of the past, but this time she was not crying—she was terrified. That night when she went to bed, she had horrible nightmares of the barn, and her grandfather standing over her. She woke up screaming. Her sister tried to comfort her, but it did not work. Soon after, her mom came into the room to see what the fuss was all about. Again, Joann remained quiet. Her mother asked about the dream, but she did not say a word, only whimpering and shaking.

Her mom rubbed her back and said, "Sleep Joann, you are safe."

Over the next few weeks, Joann became distant, depressed, and anxious. She would sit on the back steps in the hallway and rock feverishly. She refused to go outside unless it was absolutely necessary, and she gave her mom a hard time about everything. These behaviors overflowed onto her innocent sister as she started to behave mean towards her—and even going as far as to pinch her at night while she was sleeping. She would also hit and kick her sister when nobody was looking. The final breaking point came when it was time to go back to her grandparents for a visit. Joann refused to go and ran into her room hysterically crying.

Rose made her way into her room totally annoyed by her never-ending antics. Rose yelled at Joann for her bad behaviors.

That triggered her to finally tell the truth—and she blurted it all out. It was there in the room that Joann confessed to her mother what had happened in the barn with her grandfather.

Rose was shocked and said to her, "Are you me telling the truth?"

"Yes mommy. I am so scared of him. Please do not make me go."

"We have no choice, Joann. We must go, but I will have your father take care of it. Just stay away from your grandfather. Do not get in his way anymore. Now get ready, we have to leave."

Joann pulled herself together, and off they went, back to the place that terrified her. As they drove, she tried to put the awfulness out of her head and was thinking about how beautiful it really was there. They could wander around freely picking berries and feeding the animals. This was the one place that she didn't mind being outside, but now her grandfather took that little piece of happiness away from her, replacing it with fear and more anxiety.

As they pulled up the long dirt driveway, you could see the apple and pear trees lining the way, with their favorite cow (affectionately named Rosie after her mother) tied to the tree eating grass. Rose hated the fact that the family named a cow after her but chose to ignore the topic. Rose had style and class so to be compared to a cow offended her, but she remained silent in her opinions.

When they all got out, the cousins came to greet them, and with an approving nod from mom, off they went to play. Joann took a second look back at her mother who encouraged her to go and said to her, "It will be fine, just play."

What Joann did not know was that her parents had a conversation about what happened in the barn, and a plan was put into motion. They spoke to the grandfather, and of course, he denied it immensely and acted completely offended. Rose could tell he was lying as she eyed him with contempt.

Rose also found out a few things that day, which were quite disturbing. She learned that there was past talk and unspoken secrets about him fondling and inappropriately touching his own daughter! She was appalled to hear this but again remained quiet about it, holding her thoughts and judgement to herself.

When they got home that night and she was tucking her girls safely into bed, she instructed both of them to never go into the barn and stay away from grandpa.

When she was asked why by her younger daughter, the response was simple and to the point, "because I said so, and you must obey me. Do you understand?"

Both girls said yes, and that was the end of that conversation. It was never brought up again. Joann once again never had the opportunity to express what she was feeling or made to understand what happened . . . and why. Her thoughts were becoming more clouded with guilt and uncertainty.

As time moved forward, her paranoia, anxiety, and depression worsened. She would do many odd things and crazy rituals to sacrifice herself for any cause at hand that she was obsessing over. She would sleep with no blankets on in the dead of winter, freezing herself because she felt this would help her grandmother's blindness.

This is where her self-sacrificing behaviors began to form at this time in her life. She was only ten years old. If she wasn't sacrificing for something, she would be yelling and crying, as her mood swings started to form. She struggled tremendously, especially among her peers. She was jealous of her younger sister who made friends easily, ran around the neighborhood playing, and was extremely athletic. Her sister tried to include her, but it never worked out for Joann. She was always labeled the outcast.

As all the kids ran and played, she sat on the sidelines, never engaging with anyone. Most of the other kids thought she was either weird or a snob, so they poked fun at her all the time, which usually resulted in her crying or breaking out in a fit of anger. The kids would wait for her explosions as they would laugh at her quite often. This would infuriate and embarrassed her tremendously.

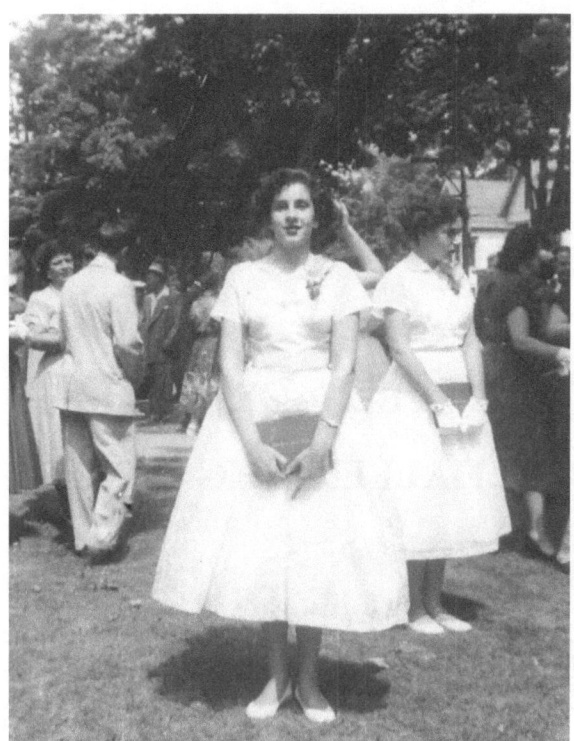
*Joann 8th Grade Graduation*

Childhood was not kind to her, and as she grew into an awkward teenager, there were changes to come. The family decided it was in the best interest for all of them to move to West Haven so they could be closer to the rest of the family. It was a hard transition for her with many growing pains, but she finally was able to settle down, making some new friends in the neighborhood.

Life was starting to look up a bit for Joann.

## Chapter 2

# The Teenage Years— Challenging Times

As a thirteen-year-old, Joann was starting to come out of her inner shell a little bit more. She began to branch out into the new neighborhood and made some friends. Joann and her sister started to hang out together which made them both happy. There were a lot of other teens that lived on their street, so there was always someone to talk to.

When they first moved to West Haven, the transition was quite difficult for her, but in time, she made peace with the move and found out she enjoyed the new environment very much. They lived in a one-family house which was gold and had two floors. She loved the look of her new home, and it was in that home that they welcomed two brothers over the next few years!

Sitting on the front porch with her best friend Anna, cousin Reena, and her sister was one of her favorite hobbies. Joann loved chewing gum, which made her feel like one of the cool kids. It was there, on that porch, that they chatted about all the new music of the '50s, the latest dance moves like the twist and the mashed potato, and *American Bandstand*. The '50s was a magical time for all teens as everything was up and coming, and they were the lucky generation to embrace it all.

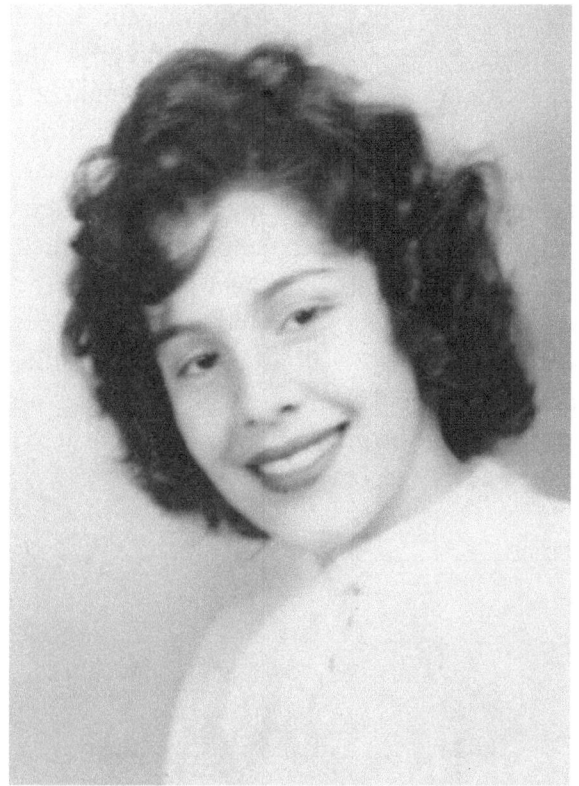

*Joann, thirteen-years-old*

It was also on that front porch that Joann met a boy who lived in the neighborhood. He would walk by the house with his friends all the time, and he would smile at her. One day he finally got up the courage to say hello, and she responded. This was the beginning of a whole new type of friendship. This young man was tall and slender with black, slicked-back hair, Elvis style. He wore a white t-shirt, jeans, and sneakers. He had soulful eyes and a bright smile.

He said to her one day, "Hey, I am John. What's up?"

"My name is Joann," she giggled.

The girls on the porch giggled as well, and a new friendship began, as this group of teens started to hang out daily.

As they all chatted over the weeks that followed, they learned so many things about each other, realizing many of them went to the same school. Joann was developing quite a feisty nature so she decided, along with her sister, to make up this crazy story to tell John.

Joann's sister had very dark skin, eyes, and hair showing her deep Italian roots that gave her these beautiful gifts. She was a dark beauty with deep brown eyes. They thought it would be funny to tell him that she was adopted, and she was an Indian (Native American). He bought it hook, line, and sinker. They laughed so hard about this, and it was a long-standing joke for years to come. They were young, beautiful, and innocent back then, embracing that true teen spirit.

As time moved forward, John and Joann began to date. They laughed together, fought together, and smoked cigarettes together. There was so much going on all around them: local dance parties, Savin Rock Amusement Park, and stock-car racing, right in their backyard, as well as the beach. These young teens had so much to do, and they enjoyed every aspect of their youth.

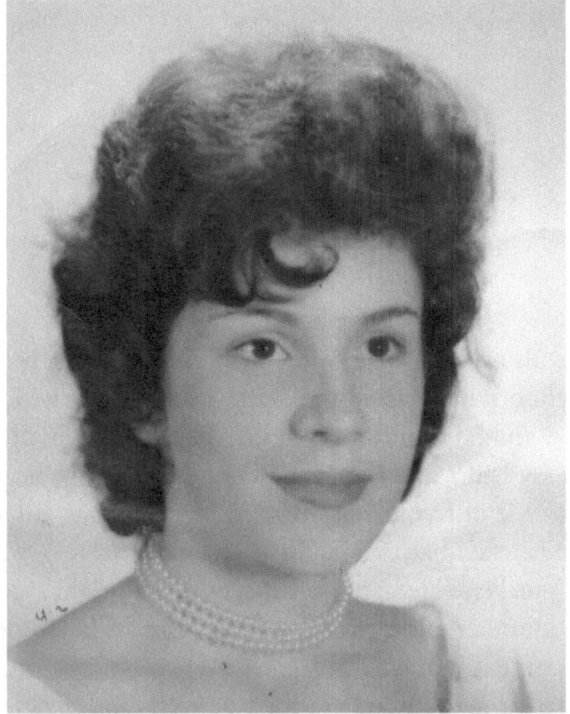

*Joann, fifteen-years-old*

It was during this time, that Joann began to struggle tremendously with anxiety and some paranoia. At times she would feel exhaustion and deep depression, and then mania would set in. She would talk a mile a minute like she was on speed. She chain-smoked to help calm her nerves. John had a very hard time understanding her mood swings and odd behaviors. They would fight like cats and dogs during these unsettling times.

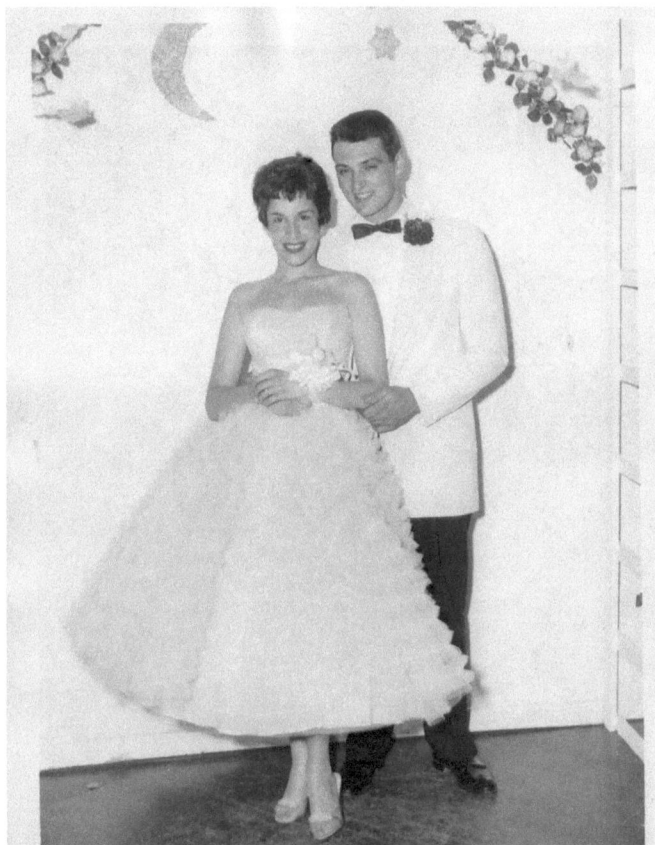

*Prom 1958*

On one occasion, he could not reach her on the phone. He redialed her number countless times only to get a busy signal over and over again. This infuriated him to the point that he drove over to her house, marching right in without even knocking. He proceeded to rip the phone right off the wall while she was talking to her friend Anna. Of course, a huge explosion happened, and this was one of the countless breakups that would occur over the course of their relationship.

They were totally in love with each other, but Joann knew how to push all his buttons as he would explode. John had a heart of gold, but a short fuse, so you can imagine this combination. They had very poor communication skills, but no matter how hard they fought, something always brought them back together.

As they made their way into adulthood, John asked for her hand in marriage, and she accepted.

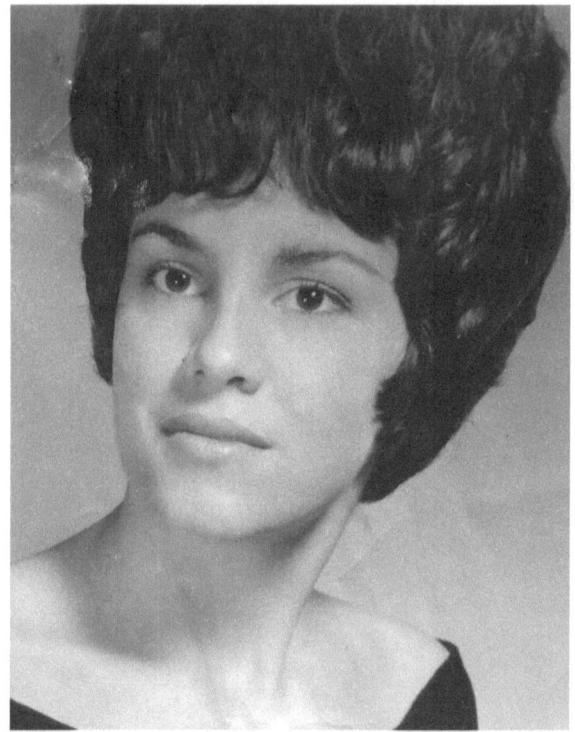

*Joann's Engagement Picture*

As the wedding preparations began, Joann's nerves got the best of her. She struggled tremendously with very little understanding. She did not know how to express herself, so she would display fits of anger, followed by endless tears. With the date closing in on her, she had much self-doubt and fear, with no clear resolve from anyone. She tried to talk to her mother who would always say to her, "Joann, be strong. You can do it."

Her sister offered kindness and urged her to move forward. Joann was scared to leave her mother, her home, and her family. She was terrified of being a wife and the expectations that came with it. The thought of having intimate relations was another huge fear that she carried with her right on up to the wedding date.

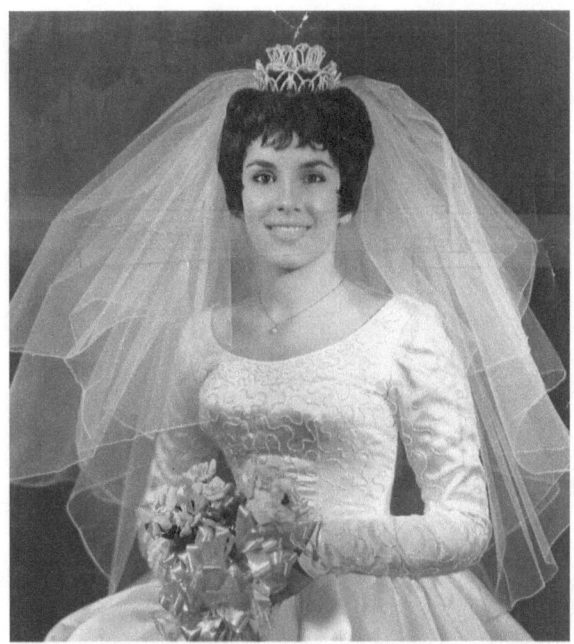

*Joann, the bride*

With constant urging, Joann made it to her wedding day filled with high anxiety, fear, and sadness. She loved John dearly, but she was consumed by these deep dark feelings that she did not understand, and she felt lost, confused by her emotions. Her past was creeping in on her, a past that she buried long ago when she moved to West Haven. She was having some flashbacks but had no clue what they were, so she tried to ignore them. She listened to her mothers' words, "be brave Joann" as she moved forward and married her childhood sweetheart.

On a cold day in November 1960, John and Joann became man and wife. They had a huge wedding with over two hundred people attending. Joann looked like a fairy princess in her beautiful beaded and satin gown, hooped skirt, wearing a crown and veil. John looked like a movie star with his big broad shoulders, dashing smile, and jet-black hair. They were a stunning couple, and they looked like they stepped right out of the movies. You would think everything was perfect, but that was far from the case.

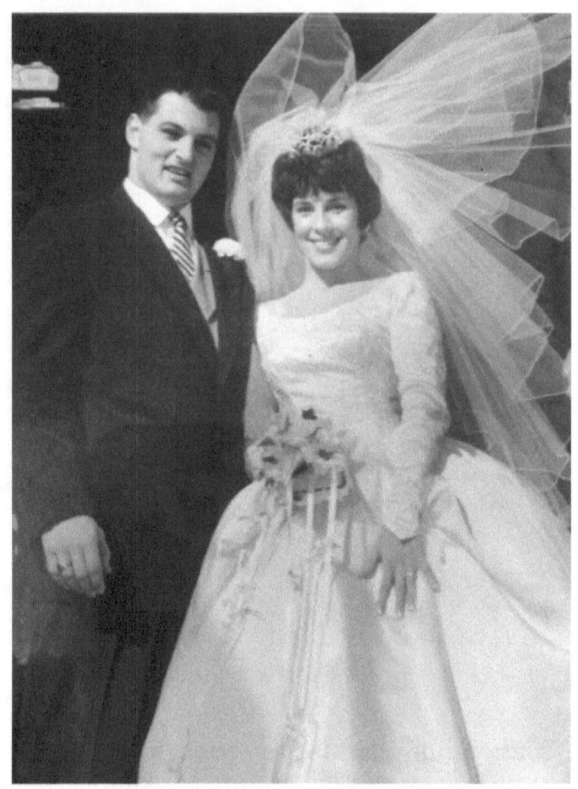

*Wedding November 25, 1961*

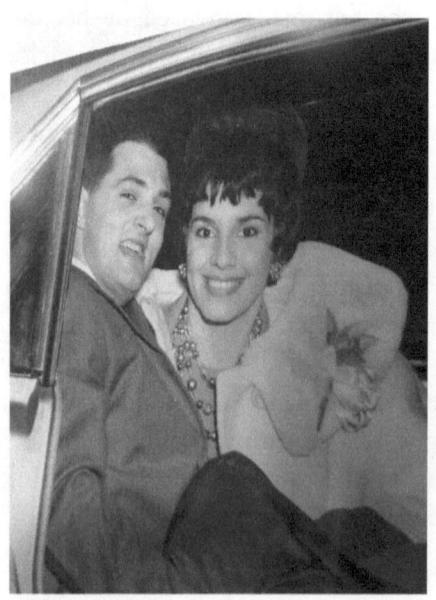

Before leaving on their honeymoon, Joann broke down crying, as she was terrified to leave her mother. As guests waited for her to make a big entrance in her honeymoon attire, she wept in the dressing room as her sister consoled her. Once again, she had to pull herself together as she stepped out with her husband in tow, smiling and waving to the crowd as they departed.

What mixed emotions she was feeling that day. The past and present were silently churning inside of her, trying to claim her ultimate joy. This should have been one of the happiest days of her life, but that was far from the case. The reality was that it was marred by the darkness of her illness that nobody acknowledged or talked about—not even her.

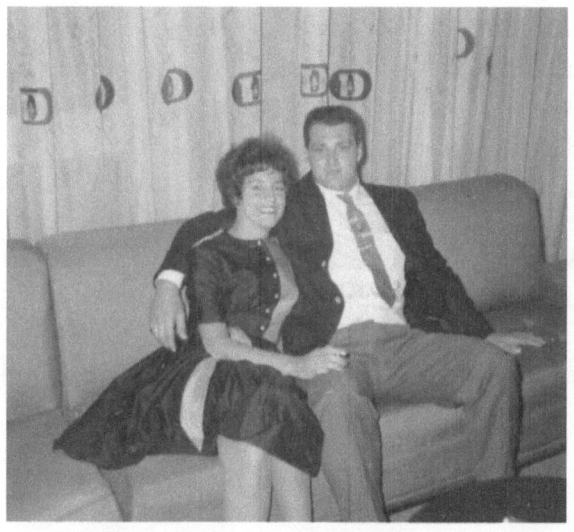

*Joann and John on their Honeymoon in Miami Beach*

After the honeymoon, they came home to West Haven and bought a beautiful new three-bedroom home. They seemed to have the perfect life being newly married, living in a beautiful home with a huge yard.

John was a grocery store manager, and Joann a hairdresser. She had great talent and was sought out by all the elite woman of stature and money. Joann worked at a lovely shop in Milford, Conneticut, and she had a huge following. You would think she would be the happiest woman in the world! It was the '60s, and all that she had achieved to this point was big back in the day, but the truth was she was very depressed. What many people did not know about her was that she struggled in every aspect of her life. Sometimes just getting out of bed was excruciating for her. Joann hid most of it well and played the part of doting wife, high fashion hair-dresser, and loyal daughter. She wore many masks, as nobody saw the reality of what she was going through.

Unfortunately, her insides were screaming for help, slowly sucking her up into an abyss of sadness. She fought hard every single day to get beyond these dark-seated thoughts and feelings. Most days seemed like a blur to her as she would go on auto-pilot robotically making her way through her days.

Then one day, while sitting on the couch after a long day of work catching up with her husband, he asked her if they could have a baby and create a family together. Joann instantly began to cry. John held her so tight thinking these were tears of joy, but that was a misguided thought on his part. She was actually terrified of becoming pregnant and being a mother. She did not feel like she was capable of doing any of it. Joann had very low self-esteem and always doubted herself worth and abilities. She had so many talents, but mental illness robbed her of that important insight.

She never expressed her feelings to her excited husband that night, but simply said, "Yes, John. Let's have a baby."

# Chapter 3

# Here Comes the Children

As time moved forward, this beautiful couple was working harder than ever. John would not only work at his full-time job, but he would moonlight at his family's seafood restaurant on nights and weekends.

After work, Joann would meet him there and sit in her favorite booth drinking diet soda, eating her clam strips (which was her favorite), and smoking. She would watch her husband work behind the counter as she would get lost in thought. The waves of anxiety would flow over her like a tidal wave, and she would shake when lighting up the next cigarette, puffing so deeply as to consume every ounce of nicotine. Her eyes would grow big and intense as she puffed away.

"Joann, Joann. Hello, can you hear me?"

As she was pulled back into reality, her husband was standing in front of her looking annoyed that she was oblivious of his presence.

"What the hell are you doing?"

"I am tired, John!"

As he sat down next to her to eat dinner, she watched him with sad eyes. Nothing in life made her happy, and she was feeling empty inside. John started to talk to her about his day and all that was going on at work. He felt pride in himself as he shared with his young wife, feeling she was hanging on every word he was saying.

She would appropriately smile at him during the right moments of the conversation, but inside she was hearing garble! It was a muffled noise of distorted voices, not only his but others. She would try to stay focused, but these other voices were calling her, and her mind was fighting an internal battle that nobody could see. When John was done eating, he got up, kissed her on the forehead, and went back to work.

Just as he turned to walk away, Joann called out to him, "John, I am going home. I am so tired and need to go to bed."

With an era of sadness in his eyes, he responded, "Ok Joann, see you at home later." He knew that by the time he got home, she would be out cold, so he immersed himself back into his work.

This was her cue to go, as she put out her cigarette, slurped the last of her soda, got up and quickly made her way out the door. She felt like she was in a clouded bubble as she rolled along not knowing which end was up. The voices were becoming louder and when she got in the car, she held her head tight, saying to herself, "Stop it, Stop it, Go Away I hate you, leave me alone."

As she violently shook her head, the tears started running down her face. She hears distorted laughter and begins to scream! Now fear turned into anger, as she started the car and aggressively dropped it into reverse, backing out without even looking. Then she kicked the car into drive pressing her foot on the gas aggressively, taking off like a bat out of hell. She flew home like a raving manic, talking and crying the whole way.

Joann finally made it home. She quickly got out of her car, slamming the driver's door and proceeded to run quickly into the house. She did not want the neighbors to see her so upset. As she made her way inside, she dropped to the floor, weeping so uncontrollably that her body began convulsing.

As she looked to the ceiling, she screams up to the universe, "Why, Why, Why am I like this? Help Me please! Help Me!"

As the room begins to spin, she continues to weep until there is nothing left. Her lifeless body sprawled out on the cold tile floor; she can barely move but eventually pulls herself to her feet. As she reached for her pack of cigarettes, her hand shakes, but she manages to strike a match lighting it. As she puffs away, she feels a release of a calm wave coming over her body. Eyes closed, puffing and puffing slowly blowing the smoke from her lips, she is finally feeling peace.

Once she is calm enough, she goes to bed and lays down on the soft cotton sheets. Feeling the coolness, she begins to relax a bit more, closing her eyes and enjoying the breeze coming through the window. She is floating. As she dozes off, she hears a voice calling out to her—soft at first, but then getting louder and louder. These strange voices start to tell her all sorts of things, and she would do her best to ignore them.

As she is laying there, she hears a door close in the distance. John had made his way home early, hoping to spend some time with his wife, catching her before she falls asleep.

The voices are whispering to her to call out a side of her that was not her, a very raunchy sexual side, one that confused her, even scared her. As John made his way into the room, there was his wife laying on the bed waiting for him.

"Joann are you awake?"

"Yes, John. Come make love to me like you never have before. I want you NOW!" she responds in a sultry voice (one that was not hers).

He was shocked but moved quickly as he wife never spoke to him that way before, and he was instantly excited. They made love all night long, wild and carefree. She would not let go, and this sexual experience was one like no other! Joann became a sex kitten pouncing on him repeatedly. She could not be tamed, nor did she want to be. When it was finally over, they both lay silently together bodies intertwined.

As John fell happily asleep, Joann rolled over, and the voices in her head called her a "Whore" over and over again. She silently cried herself to sleep.

Over the next few months, this became a cycle for Joann, going from one extreme to another, as she rode the rollercoaster of mania to the depths of depression. She was struggling but kept it hidden under the mask of a dutiful wife. Joann was trying to find understanding and balance but could not seem to figure out what was going on. She would fight those voices every day. Then as she became more tired, she noticed her body was feeling quite different. She did not understand why.

You see, Joann had a body most woman would die for, and all men wanted. She was very slim with an hour-glass figure. Her waist was only twenty-two inches, and she knew how to carry herself, standing tall sashaying as she walked. Everyone took notice of her exquisite beauty and electric smile. Joann started to notice her clothing was getting a bit tight and her tiny waist started to expand. She was perplexed. Then she became violently sick at work one day, throwing up in the staff bathroom. She came out of the door to find her boss standing there waiting for her.

"Joann are you pregnant?" her boss asked her.

"I have no idea."

She ran out of work crying hysterical. She jumped into her car and went straight to her mother's house. She burst through the door yelling, "Mom, Mom. I am pregnant. Where are you?"

Her mother came down the hallway.

"Joann, what are you doing here? Aren't you supposed to be at work?"

"I am sick, and I am pregnant." Joann begins to cry.

Her mother comes over and hugs her.

"This is wonderful news."

Joann did not feel good about any of it. She did not want to get fat, she did not want to give birth, and she was terrified of being a mother. As all these thoughts were burning through her brain, the only thing that she could say to her mom was, "John will be so happy."

Rose instructed her to call the doctor and take a test to confirm the news. Joann did as she was directed, and off she went. She went home and did not say a word to John. She was not ready to tell him the news.

The next day she got a phone call at work, and just as her boss stated, Joann was pregnant with her first child. There were such mixed emotions as she finished out her shift in a daze. She drove home and waited for her husband. She cooked him a beautiful dinner that evening and that is when she shared the news with him.

"John, it looks like you got your wish. I am pregnant. We are going to have a baby!"

He was so ecstatic, picking up his beautiful bride, twirling her around, kissing her passionately, and expressing his undying love for her.

"You did it, Joann. You, did it!"

As she rested her head on his shoulder, many things went through her mind, but she pushed it all away because she wanted to enjoy the moment.

On March 17, 1963, John Patrick arrived into the world, kicking and screaming after a very long labor and delivery. Joann felt relief that it was finally over because throughout her pregnancy she was paranoid that her baby would die. She thought about it all the time. Her anxiety level was off the charts.

When John Patrick "Jon Jon" finally arrived, he was beautiful and healthy. They were a happy little family. Joann was exhausted from her delivery and wanted to rest. She decided she did not want to see the baby for a long time.

Finally, the nurse said to her, "I am bringing you the baby. You must hold him."

She was so scared to hold him, and in the back of her mind, she had a fear that something would be wrong with him. As the nurse came in the door holding her bundle, John cried tears of joy.

"Joann, we have a son, a beautiful son! I cannot believe it; you gave me the best gift in the world."

Joann smiled and cried as the nurse handed him to her. She cuddled and rocked him for a bit. Then she kissed him on his perfect button nose, and handed him to her ecstatic husband.

"Here you go Daddy."

He took the baby out of her arms, smiling brightly, and ran up and down the hallway yelling, "Look at my son! Look at my son!" He handed out cigars to everyone, as he cried more tears of happiness. John was on top of the world at this very moment as he proudly showed off his son.

The next day the doctor came in to share some upsetting news. Joann sat up straight in her bed, waiting with bated breath of what would come out of his mouth next. The doctor stated the Jon Jon had a hernia and a testicle that did not drop. They needed to do surgery on him to fix the issue.

Joann went into hysterics and began to scream at the doctor, "My son is going to die. My son is dying."

The doctor tried to calm her down assuring her that this was routine, and he would be ok, but nothing could soothe her. He called in the nurse who quickly gave her a shot of valium to calm her hysteria. As she lay back down, she wept into her pillow, soaking it with all her pent-up fears. The doctor and nurse left her alone. When she felt up to it, she called her husband to share the news. He was already back at work as he was a workaholic. He dropped everything and came to the hospital to be by her side and his son. The doctor came back in to speak to both of them, explaining what would need to happen next. Joann mumbled to herself wanting her mother. She turned almost childlike under the stress and pressure.

John called her mother and sister to come help, and they all waited as little Jon Jon was taken into surgery. After much agonizing, worrying and a river of tears, he came out of surgery with flying colors. The doctor reported to them that their son would be perfectly fine.

John asked to see his son, and the doctor led him to the recovery area. Joann's mother and sister stayed by her side, consoling her and encouraging her to see her son.

"No," Joann said.

She just laid there in a zombie-like state for a long period of time, and then she fell asleep. Later that evening, she finally built up the courage to hold her baby boy, and she fell in love. His big brown eyes staring up at her, his pouty lips and round face. He had beautiful pink cheeks and a perfect nose! She softly sang to him, rocking him gently as he seemed to smile. He had jet black thick hair, and all the nurses made a big fuss over him. He was the "golden child" of the nursery, and Joann finally felt some pride, as she shooed away the evil voices when they popped up. This was her moment, and she was claiming it.

Finally, this little family was able to go home and begin a new stage in their lives. Joann struggled the first few months with major depression (Post-Partum), but back in the day they called it, "the baby blues."

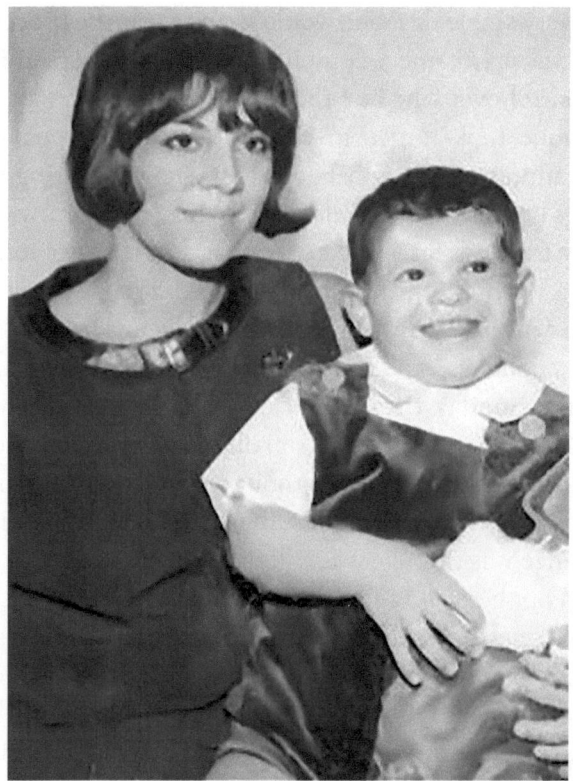
*Joann and Jon Jon*

Her sister and mother came to help, as her husband went right back to work. Joann quit her job to be a stay-at-home mother but found it to be extremely difficult. She felt isolated from the world, so her depression grew deeper. There were times Jon Jon would be in the crib screaming, but she would not go to him. She would just sit smoking her cigarettes one after the other ignoring his cries. It was a very dark time for her.

As the months passed, Joann started to feel a bit more like herself and was engaging a bit better with her son. She was neurotic about cleanliness in her house and her baby, so she went from majorly depressed to a bit manic and high strung. When she wasn't caring for the baby, she would be cleaning profusely. She would even scrub the kitchen floor tiles with a toothbrush on her hands and knees. Then she would scrub the walls, cabinets, and anything else that seemed worthy. Nothing ever felt clean enough for her, so she kept on cleaning every single day. She would even repeat the process over and over again, as it became a compulsion. This was something she felt she had control over. She had the ability to keep everything spotless.

Everyone took notice to her up and down behaviors, but it was never addressed. They believed that she was getting better with her anxiety because she was always moving. Her family and friends mistakenly took her fast-paced energy as a sign of her feeling better, instead of a warning sign of what was to come.

Time was going by, and they would engage in many family gatherings, holidays, and summers up at her mother and father's house. Every Sunday they would divide their time between John's family and hers. The family was starting to grow as her sister married and had a baby boy. It seemed as though things were moving along in life, and Joann was coping the best that she could. What many people did not realize was that she was still battling her inner demons, and it would seep out here and there, but again nobody would acknowledge it or ask the questions. She was just "Joann."

Once again, Joann shared the news with her husband that they were expecting their second child. He was thrilled that their family was growing. Jon Jon was doing well and thriving. John felt life was perfect! Joann on the other hand silently contemplated pregnancy and motherhood, as the old fears were creeping back in as her swollen belly grew. Her second pregnancy was a big struggle for her, but she made it to the end.

On November 30, 1965, Lisa Rose came into the world with a fury!

When they announced "It's a Girl," Joann's eyes lit up, and when they placed her daughter on her chest, she looked at her mother with these huge bright blue eyes just staring at her. Joann was so surprised to see these blue eyes looking at her. They were as blue as the sky. She felt some happiness, seeing this sweet face looking up at her with jet black hair.

When they handed John his little girl, he once again cried and made his way out into the hallway sharing his beautiful baby daughter. He made jokes about how loud she was!

"She is the loudest baby that I have ever heard."

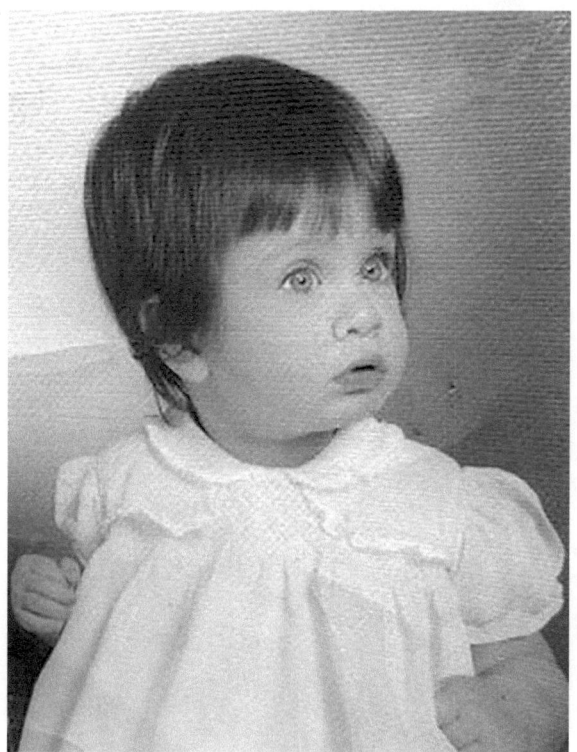

*Lisa 9 Months Old*

It was a joyful moment for these young parents. They sat in the room with their new baby girl, and John's parents brought Jon Jon to the hospital to meet his sister. He was so excited to see her. He held her tightly and kissed her tiny head.

"I love you Lisa," Jon Jon said, as everyone smiled and laughed together.

This was a precious moment in time that they all felt true happiness. Joann's incredible little family of four was about to embark on many new adventures together. They could never have foreseen the darkness and tragedies that lay ahead for them. This perfect moment frozen in time, tattooed on the hearts of these loving parents as they vowed to love and protect these two children always.

Life has a way of playing awful tricks on the unknowing victims it claims along the way. In time there will be many changes to come, and countless tears to be shed.

"Hold a moment of time in the palm of your hand, guiding it to your heart, keeping it forever safe . . . " Lisa Zarcone

# Chapter 4

# Time Marches On

As the December winds blew and the excitement of Christmas was all around, Joann relished in the holiday magic. This was the first Christmas for baby Lisa, and Joann wanted it to be special for all of them as a family. She made everything grand from the trimming of the tree, to decorating the house, and baking elaborate cookies and cakes. Joann was a fabulous cook who loved to create new and exciting meals for her family.

At Christmas time, she was best known for her Holiday Fruit Cake and Christmas Cake with Rum. On Christmas Eve, it was the Feast of the Seven Fishes and homemade Italian bread with more wine to be poured than one could possibly drink. Christmas day was her favorite because Joann and her family spent the day at her parent's home up on the hill. Everyone would gather as this growing family was extending to a new generation of children.

The tree was overloaded with presents, and there was more food than you could imagine! The antipasto was as tall as the sky, and the Christmas ham could feed an army. Tis the season!

The month of December was always her favorite because her mind was occupied with these upcoming festivities that warmed her heart. Joann was a true lover of family, and the glowing look on her face showed it.

The hardest part for her was that underneath that glow, she was battling an internal war inside her mind. One that would go on day and night with no start and no end. She would keep pushing it away, engrossing herself into the holiday, marching on like a vigilant soldier refusing to give up or wave the white flag of defeat!

Joann made it through the holidays like a victorious captain claiming her stake high upon the hills shining ever so bright. Everyone around her now felt that her past anxiety and depression was over and done, because looking at her, she was thriving as a wife and new mother of two young children. How could there be anything but joy!

The family consensus was . . . The worst was over

*Oh, mental illness what a deceitful game you play! The masking of sanity in this insane game of twisted thoughts, clouded images, and multiple personalities!*

\* \* \*

With the holidays safely tucked behind them, life became a new normal. John went back to working long extended hours, and Joann was left home alone to care for her two young children.

January arrived with the great bearer of depression. It was like a bomb that has exploded, and Joann was once again so depressed she could barely move. The days were becoming a blur to her as she was trying to cope. She was also struggling with the mania, the highs and lows rapidly cycling all around her.

With the winter snow now falling, so did the tears. Many, many tears of sadness, as the voice of "the beast" whispered in her ear: "You do not deserve to live. Die Joann Die."

Joann was distraught by the voices that continued to follow her throughout her days, as she was trying desperately to enjoy her babies. She was sinking lower and lower, and nobody seemed to notice. On the outside, she was going about her days cleaning, cooking, and taking care of the children.

Her house was spotless, so how can she be depressed?

She was also losing all of her baby weight, and she was becoming skinny once again. So how can she be depressed? Her loving husband would come home to a perfectly cooked meal filling his belly, sharing his day with his beautiful doting wife.

So how can she be depressed?

*Do you get the theme that is going on here?*

Joann hid it all well for a long time until she started to falter. She began to slow down a bit as she would fight the highs and lows of her emotions. She started to show signs of cracking. She was now losing focus on her mission and was being drawn to the voices that were singing psychotic lullabies in her head. As she listened intently, she would float away to another dimension, almost like an outer body experience. Her eyes would glass over with a blank stare.

As she floated mindlessly, the voices were telling her to ignore her children, that they were no good for her, do not acknowledge them.

In the background, Joann could hear a faint cry of her baby girl and a small voice saying, "Mommy, mommy, Lisa is crying. Why won't you answer me? Mommy, please answer me. I am scared!"

As Jon Jon started to whimper, he did not know what to do, so he started poking his mother, slow at first and then feverishly. All of a sudden, Joann jumped up, snapping back into reality, pushing Jon Jon to the floor, charging into the baby's room, and scooping Lisa up in her arms as she screams out loud.

"I am sorry, so so sorry. Please stop crying. My head, my head! Please stop crying."

She was now rocking Lisa in an almost out of control motion as Jon stood in the doorway, looking at her in horror.

"Mommy, Mommy, stop, you are hurting my sister."

Joann stopped, and Lisa began to settle down. Joann looked at her terrified son and said, "Don't ever poke me like that again. Do you hear me?"

He looked down at the floor and mumbled, "I'm sorry."

Joann then put the baby back down in the crib and turned around patting Jon Jon on the head and said, "That is my good boy, mommy loves you."

And she walked back into the kitchen to light up a cigarette.

Jon walked over the crib with tears in his eyes and whispered, "It's ok Lisa. I will protect you." He then reached in and held her tiny little hand in his, knowing that he needed to be the one to keep her safe.

When Jon walked back out of the room, Joann called him over. Now calm as a cucumber as the chemicals shifted back to normal, she had a conversation with him.

"Come sit on mommy's lap."

He is apprehensive at first, not knowing what to expect, but she is back to her loving nature with a warm smile as she swoops him up into her arms. She kisses his forehead and says, "You know mommy loves you more than anything in the world, right?"

He nods his head, and she goes on to tell him that she is the best mommy in the world but sometimes she gets tired, and he may have to be a big boy and help her with the baby. He again nods his head, silently listening to every word.

"Come on, let us color together!" Joann then says to him.

Jon Jon smiles at her and runs to grab his coloring book and crayons, and Joann thinks to herself, *What am I doing? I can't do this.*

Her heart silently breaks because she realizes what her behaviors will do to her children.

When Jon returns, they happily color together as Joann's mind wanders again. The voices are chanting her name. She fights them off so she can give her son this moment that was meant for just the two of them.

"I love you Jon Jon," she says to him.

"I love you too Mommy."

* * *

As time marches on, it is becoming harder to hide her mood swings. Her husband and mother are becoming very aware of her odd behaviors. During a family gathering, John pulls Joann's sister aside and has a conversation about his wife's behaviors. He asks her if she would check in on Joann while he was at work, and she agreed.

Joann was now in a deep depression and did not want to leave the house, but her mother would call her and say, "let's go shopping together." She would never refuse her mother, so she would pull herself together, pack the kids up in the car, and speed off to get her mom. Joann had a lead foot when it came to driving, and when she was in her manic states, she would drive quite reckless, even with the children in the car. Rose was very aware of how Joann was driving, even though she was blind. Her other senses felt what her eyes could not see.

"Joann, slow down. You're all over the road," Rose would exclaim!

Joann did as she was told, silently cursing her mother for reprimanding her.

Between her mother and sister, they did their best to keep a close eye on her, but it was hard. John worked continually, and Joann was struggling more and more. Some days she would over sleep. Jon Jon would get up and wander the house, even taking Lisa out of the crib and teaching her to climb over the side. They would get into all sorts of things together from pouring cereal and milk all over the table, to eating crayons, and dumping toys everywhere.

One day Jon Jon climbed up onto the counter and took down the baby aspirin. Johnson & Johnson's Baby Aspirin were pink and tasted like candy.

Well, Jon Jon decided to eat a few, and they were so good he ate half the bottle! He then went in to wake his mother to show her the half empty bottle. When Joann woke up enough to realize what he had done, she jumped out of bed and went into panic mode. She immediately called her mother hysterically crying as her mom tried to calm her down, telling her to call the doctor's office.

She made the phone call and was instructed to bring him in right away. Joann told them she was coming now. As she looked at her son with pink residue on his mouth from the aspirin, her head was spinning.

She was thinking, *What do I do, I am not dressed, I must go!*

She was frozen for a moment, then rushed in the bedroom to throw on a shirt and pants. As she came back down the hall, she screamed at Jon Jon, "Where is your sister?"

"I don't know," was his reply, and now he was crying!

Joann was screaming at the top of her lungs, "Lisa where are you? Oh my god, where are you?"

Suddenly, she heard a little voice calling out to her, "Mommy I am in here."

She rushed over to the cabinet, opened the door, and found Lisa hiding inside.

"Why are you in here?" she demands.

In a squeaky little voice of a two-year-old, Lisa says, "I was scared."

Joann ripped her out from under the cabinet, not even acknowledging what she was saying, grabbed her son, and raced out the door. As she was shoving them in the car, the neighbor came out.

"Joann, what is wrong?"

"My son took a whole bottle of pills."

The neighbor looked at her in horror as she jumped in the car and sped away like a demon in the night.

Joann blew through two red lights, almost hit a few cars, but managed to make it there in one piece. As she was rushing the children inside, she was crying. The nurse ushered them urgently into the back, and in came the doctor who quickly examed Jon Jon. He instructed the nurse to get him some medicine so Jon could drink it.

He turned to Joann and said, "He will be alright. We are going to give him medicine to coat his stomach, but the big question is: 'where were you?'"

Before she could answer, Jon Jon piped up and said, "she was sleeping like she always does."

The doctor eyed her with annoyance.

"Do you realize it is after 11:00 a.m.? You need to be up when your children are up!"

Joann stated that she was extremely tired.

"It doesn't matter! Be up when your kids are up. It's your responsibility. Do you hear me?"

Joann said yes and packed the kids up to go back home. As they turned to leave the doctor, he added in this statement . . . "You are not being a very good mother, are you?"

Those words cut her like a knife through her soul as she was trying her hardest to be a good mother and wife. She felt like a failure. A complete failure. Once she got home and settled in with the kids, she sat down for a moment alone and the voices in her head were calling her many names.

"LOSER, BAD MOTHER, WORTHLESS, LAZY, DUMB."

As she smoked her cigarette, the voices grew louder and louder until the phone rang to break the madness.

"Hello," she answered after picking up the receiver, listening to the voice on the other end. It was her mother checking in. Her voice soothed Joann for a moment.

"Yes, mom everything is alright. The doctor gave him medicine. Ok, yes, I will call you later, bye."

As she hungs up the phone, more tears begin to flow. She feels completely broken. This is the beginning of the end.

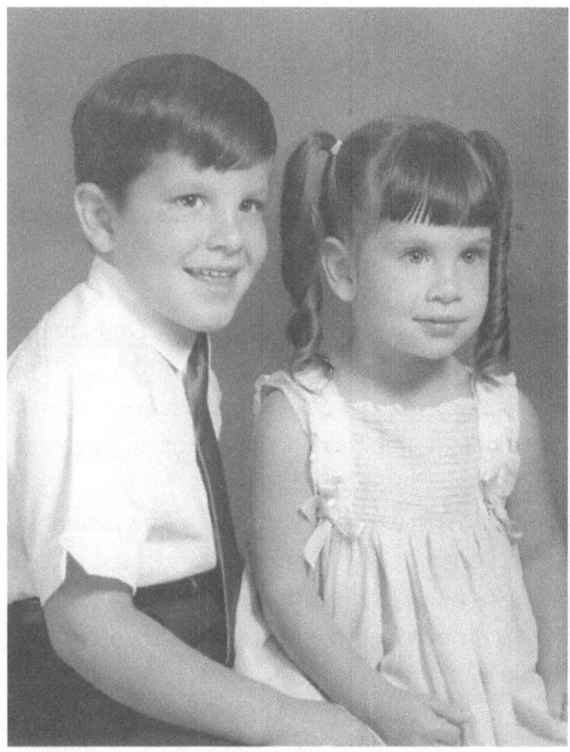

*Jon Jon and Lisa*

## Chapter 5

## The Breakdown

Over the next few months, Joann fumbled through her days feeling like she was carrying a big fish bowl on her head. Most of the time everything seemed muffled or had a long echo. The days and nights began to blend together, and it was apparent that she was struggling more than ever. She felt like she was going to totally fall apart.

As summer rolled around, her mood did lift slightly as she was around family a lot more, and the children were being monitored by other people besides her. Joann felt a bit of a break not being trapped inside that house, feeling the darkness of her obsessions. It felt good having other people help her with the children. She needed a mental health break, as it was long overdue.

In her mind, when she was home alone, she would fight the insidious voices inside her head and the continual call of duty to her children, plus the never-ending process of managing her home. She always felt that compulsive urge to scrub and scour everything in her sight. It was like a religion!

Her home never felt clean to her, so she worked feverishly trying to make it right. These behaviors were even transferred to the kids. When the kids would go outside to play and then come into the house for lunch, Joann would immediately throw them into the bathtub and scrub them down completely. Sometimes, she would scrub them so hard, not realizing what she thought was dirt, was actually a tan from the beautiful sunshine.

"Ouch! Ouch, you are hurting me. My skin is burning," her son Jon said loudly.

"Why are you not clean? Why wont the dirt come off? I must scrub more!" These were the words that would flow from Joann's mouth as her innocent children just endured what their mother was inflicting upon them. They did not know any better, so they followed their mother's lead. Joann seemed oblivious to her children's cries of pain and discomfort.

Yes, the struggle was real, as these compulsions took over her mind, body, and spirit. Joann went back on auto pilot as she listened to those voices that told her "She was worthless . . . She was an awful mother and wife . . . She did not deserve to live." Every waking moment the voices called out to her as she desperately tried to overpower them. They finally became too much for her to handle, and with the fall season upon her, she completely collapsed.

Joann would always say, "When the leaves begin to fall, everything dies and so do I. The great depression is upon us."

Joann barely made it to November with the thoughts of her daughter's second birthday pulling her forward. She was holding on to the thoughts of a big lavish party, followed by a magical Christmas.

Joann squeaked through the end of the year by the skin of her teeth!

The New Year hit with a major bang, and Joann could not take another moment. She was crawling in her own skin, as she was taunted by the madness. The mania inside her mind was on hyper-speed, and she couldn't contain her thoughts another moment.

The voices, OH THE VOICES, chanting, battling, coercing her to drop deeper into the pit of misery. "COME JOANN COME!" Joann was sitting there looking around her kitchen, eyes bulging wide open, as she puffed away on her cigarette with all her might, taking in every last ounce of nicotine.

"Go ahead Joann kill yourself, do it! It's the right thing to do. Nobody cares about you!" The voices are echoing louder and louder.

Do you hear your kids? That noise is so awfully loud. You need to get away from them—NOW!

VOICES . . . VOICES . . . THEY ARE RELENTLESS.

"COME ON FOLLOW ME TO THE DARK SIDE. YOU WILL LIKE IT HERE!!"

She had had enough. Joann jumped to her feet and screamed "STOP IT!" Then she gathered the children, packed their clothing, a few toys, necessities, and drove to her mother's house. Without any warning, they all came blasting through the door to Rose's surprise.

"Joann what are you doing here?" she asked.

Joann responded, "Mom I can't do it anymore, I cannot take care of my kids, you have to."

"What are you saying, I do not understand." Rose was shocked. Joann sent the kids into the other room, and just started screaming and crying hysterically. She couldn't stop, and her mother was scared.

"Ok, Ok, you are alright, please calm down."

Joann snorted loudly, "I cannot fucking calm down, these voices in my head will not stop taunting me! Do you hear me! AHHHHHHHHH!"

She lost complete control, and the kids came running in to see what was happening. She spun around and screamed at them to get out immediately.

"Get out of here. Do you hear me? I do not want to see either of you! Go, just go—NOW—NOW—NOW!"

Joann looked like an evil monster, and the kids were terrified. Then Jon grabbed Lisa by the hand and dragged her back into the other room, holding her tightly as they both sobbed profusely. They were shaking with fright.

Rose raised her voice to try to regain control of the scene. "Joann, go in my room right now! Do you hear me, go lay on my bed to calm down. I am calling your sister."

"Yeah, that's right. You call her. Summon the good daughter, go ahead you heartless bitch!"

Rose became agitated but ignored her, knowing what she needed to do.

After she hung up the phone, Rose tended to her grandchildren and comforted them the best she could. Rose was a soothing presence with her strong virtue. Soon Joann's sister came barreling through the door and marched straight to the bedroom.

"Joann, Joann it's me," said her sister.

"What do you want?" Joann said with a snide tone, behaving like someone else.

Her sister was perplexed as it was like she had a different personality altogether.

Joann went on to badger her sister, saying all types of mean things to her. When she was done, she dropped to the floor and sobbed. She cried for what seemed like an eternity with her sister just standing there in disbelief.

When the dust settled, her sister took her hand and guided her up as she helped her on to the bed once again.

"Joann I am going to call the doctor."

Joann, did not respond, she was now silent. The doctor instructed them to take her to the emergency room for an evaluation. They called John, who was at work, to meet them there.

As they were leaving the house, Rose said to her, "Joann, take care of you, and I will keep the children safe."

Joann looked at her mother and said, "Good because I am never coming back. I hate those brats. Those kids wrecked my life."

Joann proceeded to walk out the door without even acknowledging her babies that she loved so dearly.

As she walked on by the children, they cried, "Mommy, Mommy please don't go! Don't leave us!"

She ignored them completely. Joann was mentally gone. The daunting cries of her children were blocked by the devious voices inside her mind.

After many hours at the hospital, it was determined that Joann had had a nervous breakdown, needing to be hospitalized in the psychiatric unit.

John was in denial that there was anything wrong with his beautiful wife and began yelling at her to snap out of it. He was telling her, "You need to come home where you belong."

Joann looked at him and said "Go Fuck Yourself!"

John didn't know what to say, as he could not wrap his head around what was happening. The doctor pulled him aside and said, "She is very sick, and you cannot help her now. Leave the task to us. Remember that this is not your wife talking, it is the sickness inside her brain! Your wife has mental illness."

John stared at the doctor in disbelief.

John then reluctantly agreed and signed all the appropriate papers, and just like that, they whisked her away. She didn't even bother to look at him as they wheeled her off to what would be months of hell for both of them.

*How could this be happening?* John thought to himself, as he stood there with tears in his eyes. *My beautiful, incredible wife, sick! This is not right.*

The nurse turned to him and said, "Go home and be with your children. They need you now."

He felt defeated, angry, and confused.

*How could this happen to my perfect family. What do I do now? I don't know what to do!*

John stood there for a long time as the realization set in.

*I just lost my wife.*

# Chapter 6

# Time in the Psychiatric Unit— Hell On Earth

As they wheeled Joann upstairs, a new side of her began to emerge. She looked at the nurse walking by her side and said to her "Nice Tits Bitch!" with a wicked smile on her face.

The nurse ignored her as they moved forward. Joann was annoyed that this nurse chose to ignore her, so she decided to raise the bar a bit. "So, tell me nurse Rachet, does your pussy get any action with that nasty scowl on your face?"

The nurse turned to her and said, "Shut up!"

Joann did not like this response and without any warning, she jumped out of the wheel chair and attacked the nurse, biting and scratching her before the orderlies could pull her off. She had the strength of ten men in this moment, with daggers radiating from her eyes as she latched on for dear life. They had an extremely hard time removing her from the nurse as Joann spit in her face repeatedly. Once they finally pulled them apart, the tattered nurse sat sobbing on the floor, bleeding and disheveled. As they were dragging Joann away, she was kicking and screaming every obscenity that she could think of and more. The words rolled off her tongue as they burned her throat with twisted delight.

As the doors closed behind her with a loud BANG, she knew life was going to get quite interesting, and she was ready to play!

This was the second time in Joann's life that she spoke in such a dirty way, and the impulsive violence was not her normal behavior. During this moment, she felt like she had transcended out of her body and was watching someone else, but she felt the rush at the same time. She was two beings in one body, and it was an exhilarating experience. Joann felt more alive than ever in this moment of dysfunctional behavior, and that is where it began, that addiction to the mania.

What depths would she go to obtain that feeling again?

Joann would spend the next seven days in "Lock Up," as she called it, at the Yale Psychiatric Unit. Those seven days were filled with many harrowing moments for her, as she got a good education at what "crazy" really looked like!

Upon wheeling her into her new room, she was slouched over in the chair no longer badgering or even speaking. The adrenaline she used during the attack on the nurse had seemed to drain her of all abilities to move or speak. Then a nurse instructed her to stand as she need to undress and get naked for a cavity search.

Joann looked up at her with one eye half opened, dazed as the image of the nurse's face seemed fuzzy at first. Then she squinted to try to get a better look. Joann was trying to take in all the words that the nurse was saying to her, but it sounded extremely confusing.

Joann then felt like these words seemed to begin to burn the inside of her head, and she abruptly raised her hands to cover her ears, not wanting to take in the sounds.

"My head is burning!" she screams, "STOP TALKING!" I can't take it!" Joann began to rev up again, as the nurse tried to speak calmly to her.

The nurse instructed her again to get undressed as it was procedure. Joann was mortified at the thought of the nurse placing hands on her, checking her body, and touching her private areas. As the burning continued inside her mind, and the words were registering more and more, so did her temper.

She snapped at the nurse, "Over my dead body, will you touch me!"

The nurse responded with, "Joann please, we can do this the easy way, or we can do it the hard way."

"OH YEAH, whore, lets fight!" She jumped up from the chair ready to attack, but this time to her surprise, two male orderlies were ready for her, and they both grabbed her immediately as Joann began to panic.

Her memories of abuse were flashing before her face —seeing her grandfather throwing her to the ground exposing himself, and the man at the grocery store pulling her in the back room. Those psychedelic images, sped up with a warped sound of her tiny screams of the past, now had her feeling traumatized with fear, as something different began to transpire.

A dark image emerged from the chaos calling out to her, encouraging her to hurt everyone in her path, "Kill them!" Kill them!" Chanted the crackling voice.

Within moments, her eyes turned black as coal, and she began to fight for her life. The nurse immediately called in the doctor for assistance, who shot her up with medications to calm her down. The doctor tried speaking to her, but she was not hearing his words as she continued to scream for her life with every ounce of her being. She felt every thread of her pain of the past, coming through as she thrashed from side to side like a fish on a hook trying to break free —but then it slowly came to a stop.

As she lay there motionless in a catatonic state, the nurse proceeded to undress her, searched her, then she slapped a johnny coat on her. Next, they tucked her in bed, and the orderlies strapped her in, tying her arms to the railings.

When she woke up hours later, it was dark in the room, with only a small light coming through the window on her door. Even this little glimmer of light hurt her eyes tremendously as her head pounded. Everything was spinning, and the colors she witnessed were dancing in the stream of light. It was a dance of splendor, as her mind wandered for a bit, hearing music in the background .She tried to lift her hands in the air to clap to the beat and that was when she felt resistance.

Splendor turned to panic as she tried to move, yanking at her arms and trying to move her legs — but she was trapped. Now fear and panic set in, and thoughts of her children ran through her mind.

"They stole my children, and they are molesting them while I am tied up!"

This thought grew bigger, and bigger in her mind, and she could see it. Her babies being fondled by many different people, passed around, shared, and being abused. She could hear the cries of her children, and she was helpless.

"Help, help my children! Help my children!" Joann screamed for what seemed like an eternity, and the tears of horror began to flow.

Finally, a nurse came in, flicked on the light, and Joann winced at the brightness. She begged the nurse to untie her so she could save her children. She was in true panic mode and believed wholeheartedly that her babies were in grave danger. The nurse asked her if she knew where she was.

"I am in a prison in Jerusalem, being persecuted like Jesus, and they took my children away from me!"

The nurse was kind hearted and spoke gently to Joann, trying to guide her back to reality. The nurse untied her arms and unbuckled the restraints, to help relieve some of the anxiety and calm the hallucinations. It seemed to be working.

Finally, Joann realized where she was, and rolled over and sobbed profusely. The nurse tried to comfort her and told it would be ok. She just needed to cooperate and let them help her. She went silent and fell asleep as the tears rolled down her face, soaking the sheets.

For the next three days, Joann was silent. The doctors and nurses were in and out of her room continually trying to engage her in conversation, but she did not utter a word. She wanted to die. The thought of dying flowed through her brain, and the many images of death came to her over those three days.

She did not eat, and she barely drank anything. All she wanted to do was sleep, praying for God to take her to heaven to be with her best friend Jesus. Joann also thought about how Jesus suffered for the good of the people, and she now believed she was one of his disciples. An image came to her with Jesus holding his hands out to her, telling her, "Joann, you are my sister, and you need to suffer to save others. There will be blood on your hands for the sake of God." She saw him clear as day and even felt him touch her hand. He went on to say, "You are the chosen one, and we will travel many miles together."

Then she saw a storm brewing behind him as the clouds rose. She was now scared as she stood beside him and out of the darkness rose Satan, spewing fire and lightning at them. She turned away and wanted to run, but Jesus stopped her and said, "NO RUNNING! You must turn and face your maker!"

Joann was confused. "Maker? Jesus, I thought you were my friend!"

"You have no friends. Everyone hates you. You are worthless to the world, and you must suffer to make your peace in this life!" Then with a crack of lightening, Jesus turned into the devil. As Joann felt the horror, she began to scream.

The nurses came running in. These were the first sounds that Joann made after three days, and once again she was fighting for her life! What she did not know, was she was living in a hallucination. You see, for Joann, it was HER reality! They had to inject her with more medication to calm her down, and for the next two days, she was once again silent.

The doctor called her husband John in for a meeting. He sat nervously with the doctor as he explained to him, that his wife was severely ill and needed more extensive care. The doctor went on to tell him about a mental health facility in Middletown, Connecticut. He felt they were more equipped to handle Joann's case, and it would be the best solution for her. John didn't know what to think and was blown away, as he hoped his wife was better and ready to come home. He needed her, the children needed her, but she was mentally gone.

John brokenheartedly agreed, once again signing papers and asking to see his wife. The escorted him to her room. As he walked into the unit, he was horrified at the sight. People everywhere sitting in chairs hunched over. Many of them so drugged up, they had to be tied into their chairs. Then he heard the moaning of some, and the screaming of others. John was a big tough man, but this shattered him to the core.

As he walked into the room, there was his wife tied to the bed. He went over to her, touched her face, and said, "Joann, it's me Johnny. Can you hear me?"

She slowly rolled over and looked into his eyes and said, "Get the fuck out of here! You put me here and I will never forgive you!" She rolled back over and said quietly, "You can leave now, you are dead to me. I hate you!"

John didn't know what to say, or to do. He stood there with a blank expression on his face, then turned around and walked out the door.

As the main door on the unit slammed behind him, he broke down in tears. The pain ripped through his heart. His incredibly beautiful wife that he loved so much was gone, and she may never come back. The thought of the words that rolled from her lips, crushed his soul. The tears poured from his eyes and his anger exploded. He punched the wall over and over again as he screamed *"WHY?"?"?"*

He left the hospital that day a broken man and went home to see his children. He also decided on what arrangements needed to be made with his mother-in-law about their care. The children would live with her, while he worked. He would come visit them at night and go back to his house to sleep. It was a very chaotic time for all of them. Nobody knew quite what to do, or how to act.

Little Jon and Lisa cried for their mother, and would beg their dad not to leave, when he had to go. Rose was the backbone of the whole operation and took the lead, directing everyone as to what they needed to do. She was a strong woman, and she made sure those children were well cared for. It was scary time for all of them.

As for Joann, the day after seeing her husband, she left Yale, a destroyed woman, with no will to live. They took her to Middletown Psychiatric Hospital, where she would spend the next four months of her life. Four months of complete hell.

Would Joann make it back to her family?

Nobody had any answers.

# Chapter 7

# Middle Town Psychiatric Unit

Joann arrived at the hospital strapped to a gurney. She was fit to be tied, literally! As they took her out of the ambulance, she spewed obscenities at the EMTs who transported her on to the next leg of this psychedelic journey. The words that were rolling across her lips would make your skin crawl.

The doors opened and this new foreign place she entered inside looked dark and dingy with the feeling of death and mayhem all around. There were no smiles to greet, only stone-faced nurses and orderlies who had no time for her nonsense.

Joann screamed and tried to break free, feeling she needed to fight for her life. The only voice she heard was the nurse telling her to shut up or they would sedate her immediately.

Joann looked her in the eye and said, "You're the first one on my list. I will get you in due time you cunt!" Then she spit at her.

The nurse ignored her until they wheeled her through the doors, and with the slamming of metal, it was game on. The nurse instructed the EMTs to bring her into an exam room and transfer her onto the bed. As they did what they were told, Joann had fire in her eyes waiting to pounce as the voices in her head were screaming at her, *"Take the bitch down!"* over and over again. Her adrenaline was building, but an uneasy calm washed over her. As they unstrapped her, she willingly got off of the gurney and onto the exam table.

The EMTs left the room, and the door locked. She sat there waiting patiently to make her move. The image of choking that bitch nurse was playing out in her head repeatedly, and she revved up with secret delight.

When the door opened, the nurse returned with two orderlies and explained to her that they needed to do a physical exam, and another cavity search. Joann was steaming with fury, and without a sound or warning, she leapt off the table and gripped her hands tightly around the nurse's neck. She choked her with such detest.

The orderlies charged into action, grabbing and pulling her off the nurse. Joann refused to let go and squeezed harder. The fear in the nurse's eyes only fed her desire to continue on her mission. As she was gasping for air, Joann laughed in her facing screaming, "How do you like that bitch! That will teach you to talk to me like that, you WHORE!" Finally, they were able to pull her away.

In that moment, she again had the strength of ten men and was determined to make it last as long as possible. She fought the two men until they finally brought her down to the floor with a hard bang. Joann screamed in distress as another nurse came over and stuck her intensely with a needle. Slowly she began to deflate like a balloon losing air and things become blurred as the room spun. She spoke, but no words came out, and slowly she closed her eyes.

When she woke up, she was in a room with two other women, and the door was locked. She was groggy, confused, and disoriented. As she regained her focus, one of the women got up and sat on her bed.

"What an entrance that was," she said.

Joann replied, "What the fuck are you talking about?"

"You don't remember?" the woman asked.

Joann sat up and tried to think. Her memory, choppy at first, started to come back to her. She looked at the woman and said, "Get off my bed, now!"

"Wow, not too friendly, are you?" The woman got up, walked to the other woman, and put her arm around her. The other woman was smaller, thin, and highly drugged up. Her eyes looked sad and droopy.

"My name is Evelyn, and this is my room. What I say goes." She leaned over and started making out with the other woman, groping her lifeless body. "You understand Joann?"

The other woman looked at her with sad, tormented eyes and gave her a half smile. Joann looked at her and said, "Well Evelyn, there is a new sheriff in town, and I do not take orders from you. Just leave me be."

Evelyn was not impressed by Joann's response and went on to say there would be trouble for her, if she went against her. Joann just flashed her a look. This was a look to be feared, as the daggers of hate sizzled right through Evelyn's body. She did not know how to quite take that look, so she laughed nervously and said, "I guess this will be interesting."

"Oh yes it will," Joann stated.

As the days transpired forward, there would be more outbursts from Joann, and more wrestling matches with the orderlies. She was bruised from head to toe, but she refused to give in.

She would meet with the staff psychiatrist daily. and he discussed what medications he would be prescribing her. Joann did not want to be medicated; she liked the freedom of these feelings that she had never had before. She craved the total mania and wanted it all the time. Her thoughts were out of control, and nothing she spoke about made sense to anyone, as the hallucinations were building. She seemed to have forgotten about her children, or the life that was waiting for her beyond the concrete walls. When the doctor brought up her husband or children, she would flip out, not wanting to hear about them or see them.

Day after day, she fought the system. Her doctor would tell her how her husband wanted to come visit, and she refused him every time. They were slowly getting medicine into her system, but nothing seemed to be working. Whenever possible, she would cheek her meds and then go flush them down the toilet. She was convinced they were trying to poison her, and she played the game with them. Joann was very good at lying, manipulating the nurses, and getting her own way. She would lay in bed and contemplate her next move. It was a strategic game of mental madness, and she was becoming a professional.

The troubles continued with Evelyn and her muse as they co-existed in the same room. Many verbal battles resulted with the nurses and orderlies coming in to break it up, but they left them in the same room together as tensions continued to rise.

Joann would think to herself, *In due time Evelyn!* She would stare at her with cold dark eyes, and Evelyn would stare back.

Joann's next visit with the doctor brought a big surprise for her. As they brought her in, she saw a man standing there with his back to her, looking out the window. She recognized those big shoulders and broad back immediately; it was her husband. He turned around with a half-smile, which quickly dropped from his face. He was in shock and disbelief of what he saw standing before him. His beautiful wife, now tattered, bruised, and disheveled. She was skinny and had dark circles under her eyes.

"What's the matter John? Not liking what you see? Take a good hard look. This is your wife now, the real me!"

It took all that he had not to cry.

He walked over to her and said, "Joann, I miss you. Please come home, we need you." As he went to hug her, she pushed him away.

"Don't touch me you mother fucker! I hate you! You forced me to have sex and have children I did not want! Don't ever touch me again!"

Before John could respond, the doctor interjected and said, "Come sit down Joann. Let's just talk for a bit."

As she sat there with this crazy look in her eyes, John could not help but stare at her, trying to find his wife in there somewhere—but he could not. The doctor went on to talk to both of them and discussed other medical options to help Joann overcome her mania and "get better" as he put it.

She looked at the doctor and said, "There is no cure for me, and I like the way that I am now. Leave me alone and just let me be."

As the doctor tried to talk to her, she just started screaming at him and became enraged! John tried to calm her down, but she would not listen to anyone. She was only hearing the voices in her head demanding her to ignore them, telling her John hated her and would only harm her if she went home. Joann went completely out of control, and the orderlies had to restrain her, as John looked on in horror. As they dragged her out, she screamed at her husband, "Don't ever come back. I hate you!"

John dropped into the chair visibly shaken up by the whole experience. He turned to the doctor and said, "You need to fix my wife immediately. We need her home, the kids miss her, I miss her."

The doctor went on to talk about other options and felt that electric shock treatments to her brain would help get her back on track. As he explained it further, John stopped him in mid-sentence and said, "Do whatever you have to do to bring her back. I don't care, I want her back to the way she used to be." The doctor shook his head, and John got up and left.

Once they got Joann back into her room, she felt that burning sensation in her arm as they jabbed her with a big needle filled with what she called "dope" and off to sleep she went. She woke up hours later, and it was dark. Her head was pounding, and she felt very weak.

Joann realized at that moment Evelyn was standing over her, and before she could do anything, Evelyn grabbed her and put her hand over her mouth pinning her down. She called upon her muse Gloria to come over and give Joann the treatment.

Joann was still so drugged up she could not fight, and as Evelyn pressed down upon her tightly, she instructed Gloria to rape her. Gloria began to giggle a twisted giggle and ripped off Joann's pants, shoved her fingers deep inside of her, pumping in and out fiercely! Evelyn was licking Joann's face, grunting with excitement.

"Do you like that Joann? I know you do; your pussy is so wet! Eat it up Gloria, eat it up!" she called to Gloria.

Joann was mortified and could do nothing to fight for herself as these nasty drugs running through her veins made her paralyzed. They took turns raping her over and over again until they were finally through.

When it was over, Evelyn looked at her and said, "Who is Sheriff now?" Gloria stood behind her giggling, and they both dropped to the floor and finished each other off, as Joann laid there motionless.

The next morning Joann was back into her catatonic state of mind, numb from what happened the night before, voiceless and broken. The nurses came in and gave her her meds, and she took them, swallowing hard as she wanted them to numb the pain. In that moment, she did not want to feel anymore. It was like a bomb exploded, and she was done.

As her roommates happily went off to breakfast, Joann whispered to the nurse, "They raped me."

The nurse looked at her and said, "What did you say?"

"Those bitches raped me last night. I need to get out of here."

At first the nurse did not believe her, but as Evelyn and Gloria chatted over breakfast, they were boasting about what they did! They were immediately escorted to the office and dealt with, as Joann later heard through the grapevine. Both women were transferred to different hospitals, and the subject was never brought up again. Joann was never given the opportunity to talk about it, not even with the doctors. The incident was pushed under the carpet.

**Moving forward.**

The doctors continued current treatments, but success proved to be challenging. They finally did catch on to the fact that Joann was cheeking her medications, so they decided to give her daily injections instead. Joann went from this highly toxic mania state with hallucinations to extreme depression. The doctor ordered the electric shock treatment therapy to begin. Joann didn't know what was coming as they did not tell her ahead of time. They did not want her to know what the plan would involve.

The decision was Electric Shock Therapy (EST)—

During the 1950s and 1960s, EST was used as punishment to regain control of patients who were not compliant. If you remember the movie *One Flew Over the Cuckoo's Nest*, there are scenes in there that show this sort of treatment towards unruly patients.

Now they call this treatment—Electroconvulsive Therapy (ECT)

Electroconvulsive therapy is a procedure done under general anesthesia, in which small electric currents are passed through the brain intentionally triggering a brief seizure. ECT seems to cause changes in the brain chemistry that can quickly reverse symptoms of certain mental health conditions. This can lift depression in some patients as it corrects nerves that have "short circuited." This treatment also changes levels of dopamine, norepinephrine, and serotonin which play roles in depression. Memory loss can occur after treatment, but in most cases it is temporary. Studies have shown it does help with acute mania.

**Let the treatment begin.**

On the day of her first treatment, they took her down a long hallway, far away from where the patients were held. As they wheeled her down the dark corridor, she began to panic a bit and asked where they were taking her. The nurse explained it was a new treatment that would make her better.

"I do not want a new treatment," Joann responded.

The nurse said to her, "The doctor ordered it."

They wheeled her into a room with no windows. Gadgets and machines were everywhere. With a full view, Joann saw a table in the middle of the room with many straps.

Joann began to cry, saying "No, No! Don't hurt me! Please I will be good, don't hurt me." Joann was brought back to childhood in her mind, and all of her fears were flooding her body. As fear turned into panic, she began to fight, and the orderlies quickly grabbed her, dropping her on the table and forcefully strapping her to it.

As the tears began to flow, there was no sympathy, explanation of any kind, or support. They all stood there silently like statues, as Joann was terrified for her life.

The doctor came in next and said, "Joann this is for your own good, do not fight it."

They prepared her for the treatment, putting electrodes on her head and body. The doctor simply explained to her that they were going to shock her brain to help get her back to "NORMAL."

Joann was stuck. She could not fight anymore, as the straps were so tight that she couldn't move. She gave up! Joann closed her eyes and endured the horrible pain that was inflicted upon her. She was supposed to be put into a twilight sleep, but she was very aware of what was happening to her. Over and over again, they shocked her brain. As she felt each zap, tears continued to flow. These were tears of blame, shame, resentment, and horror.

When it was over, they took her back to her room to rest. This time she was alone in her room. No more roommates. Joann was grateful for that. As she lay there staring up at the ceiling, she heard music. She began to hum as she watched little angels dance before her on the ceiling. She was smiling as they smiled back.

Then the angels turned into small children, and they began to cry. Joann cried too. As she reacheded up to console them, the cries became louder.

She mumbled, "My babies. Jon Jon and Lisa, mommy is here, I am here please don't cry!"

Joann now saw images in her head of her two children. She rolled over and wept until she fell asleep.

As she was drifting off, she told herself, "I must go home to my babies. They need me. John my loving husband, I am so very sorry."

# Chapter 8

# Transition Back To The Real World

After almost five months from being away from home, Joann finally felt ready to leave the hospital. She had many mixed emotions and fears about going home, but she knew that she needed to get back to her family. She did miss them all very much. As the medications finally took effect, she came back down from her mania only to transfer her emotions toward depression. Joann cried all the time and felt emotionally weak and fragile. She explained her fears to the doctor who encouraged her to move forward and to continue outside counseling, and group therapy.

He stressed to her that it was very important to take her medications every day, and to not miss a dose. She promised him that she would take care of herself.

As she sat there nervously, her mind began to wander.

*Will I be able to take care of my children? Will I be able to fulfill all of my duties as a wife? My mother needs me because of her blindness. Will I be able to help her?*

So many questions were rolling inside her mind. Joann was twitching in the chair like a child impatiently waiting for something to happen.

A knock on the door snapped her back into reality. The nurse escorted her husband in, and he came right over to her and wrapped his arms lovingly around her saying, "Joann, I missed you so much, and I am so happy that you are coming home."

She hugged him back, but she felt completely numb. All of the feelings that she had for him prior to this experience, had changed inside of her in so many ways. She gave him a half smile, but inside her mind she was confused and pondering her lack of emotion for this man that stood before her. The love of her life. Big John as they called him. Strong and extremely handsome. She secretly prayed that the feelings would come back to her. She briefly asked about the children, and he excitedly told her how they cannot wait to see her and go back home.

That word "HOME" instantly terrified her. She looked at him and said, "We are going home? I thought we were going to my mother's house? I cannot go home and be alone with the kids, not yet!"

John looked perplexed and shot the doctor an angry glare.

"I thought you said she was ready to come home. What the hell is this all about"?

Joann looked at him in terror, but before she could speak, the doctor interjected and simply stated, "John your wife needs to transition back to the house and all of her duties that come with it in a slow fashion. So, it is reasonable for her to want to stay at her mother's house for a bit to have extra support before going home to handle all of the responsibilities alone."

John shot a look at Joann and said, "OK, whatever is best."

Joann could feel the tension and became scared of him.

"I am not sure if I can go home now." Joann stated.

John looked at her and said, "Well, you do not have a choice ,let's go."

With that blunt statement being made, the doctor turned to Joann and urged her to go home. He promised her it would be all right. Reluctantly, she moved forward, and before she knew it, she was out the front door breathing in fresh air. It felt so wonderful that she stopped for a moment to take it all in.

"Why are you stopping?" John asked.

"Do you realize I have not been outside of these walls in months?" Joann replied.

He looked at her and the realization set in, and he gave a heavy sigh. "It really is a beautiful day outside. Let's go to your mother's house and see the kids, they are anxiously waiting for you."

"Ok, let's go. I think I am ready now."

As she got into the car, John closed the door for her and got into the driver's seat. He reached for her hand, and she took it. As they drove away, she stared back at the hospital half wishing she was still behind those walls so she could hide away from the world.

John put on the radio and played some music which seemed to lighten the mood as she hummed along to the beats. Joann started to relax, and she almost felt a bit excited to see everyone. As they pulled into the long dirt driveway, she could see the kids in the yard running around playing. Her mom was sitting under the large weeping willow tree wearing her big straw hat.

Once the kids heard the car pull in, they stopped what they were doing, and started screaming, "Mommy is home! Mommy is home!" They ran toward the car as Joann got out.

This was the first time she had seen her babies in months. She bent down, and they both wrapped their arms around her embracing her so tightly.

Jon Jon said, "Mommy we missed you so much. Please don't ever leave us again!"

"I won't leave again, I promise."

Those words were bittersweet for Joann, but they also cut her heart like a knife at the same time. This was because she loved them so much and was feeling that she may not be able to hold up her end of the bargain.

Lisa was clinging on to her mom but remained silent. Joann looked at her, giving her a warm smile and said, "Did you miss your mommy?"

Lisa nodded her head yes, seeming to be a bit apprehensive and scared of her. Then like a flash, she turned around and ran to her grandmother for security, clinging tightly onto her leg. Joann looked extremely sad and disappointed.

John turned to her and said, "She will be fine. It has just been a very long time since she has seen you."

Joann nodded but felt that ping of pain inside of her heart.

Rose walked over with Lisa in tow and hugged her daughter briefly. "You look good Joann. Let's go inside so we can have a cup of coffee and talk."

That was the best thing that Joann had heard in a long time. She loved her coffee and knew that she would be able to sit and smoke at the same time.

As they were making their way into the house, Rose said, "Don't worry about Lisa. She will come around. It's been kind of hard for her without you. Jon Jon has been a huge help taking care of her for me."

Joann responded, "That's good. He is a good boy."

As they all sat around the table chatting, it became slightly easier as the kids were now doting on Joann. They made her many beautiful pictures, and Lisa picked a flower for her from the yard. She handed it to her mommy with a half smile. Joann began to cry.

"No more tears Joann, be tough," Rose said.

Joann looked at her, wiped her tears, and before she knew it, the day was over. They put the kids to bed and made a plan as to what would transpire over the next few days.

It was decided Joann and the kids would live at her parents' home for a week and then transition back to their home. John would go back and forth between work, his in-laws and home. Over the next few days many visitors came to greet Joann back into the real world. This made her feel a bit stronger with so much help coming from the family. Her sister came every day to support Joann. The week flew by quickly, and the anxiety was slowly building as it was getting near her time to go back home.

Joann called her doctor to discuss her feelings, and once again he reassured her it would be ok. He directed her to the therapist that was set in place for her and told her that she needed to set up appointments immediately. The local mental health office was not far from where they lived, so it would not be hard for her to get there; except she had now developed a fear of driving because she had been away for so very long. With more coaxing and encouragement from her mother and the doctor, she agreed to drive to the office. She would take the children to her mother, see the doctor, and pick them up afterward.

She felt over-whelmed by the thought of all of it, but she kept her fears to herself. She just agreed to what everyone was telling her to do.

The next day John came up to the house to claim her and the children. It was time to bring them back home to Wildwood Terrace, a place that she truly loved at one time.

As she hugged her mother tightly before leaving, she said to her mom, "I do not want to leave you."

"It is ok Joann. you can do this." Rose stated. "Now go, be with your family, they need you."

As John stood there waiting for her, she slowly made her way to the door and walked to the car. She took a deep breath as she got in and closed her eyes as they pulled out of the driveway. The kids were in the back seat, so excited to finally be going home. They were laughing and giggling —and Joann felt sudden doom. When they pulled up to the house, she was completely terrified to step back into her duties as a wife and a mother. She knew once inside those doors, it would be game on.

She thought to herself, *"I cannot do this. Why is God punishing me like this?"* She wanted to cry!

John came around to her side of the car and opened the door, helping her out

The neighbor Ella, who lived next door, joyfully yelled out of her kitchen window, "Welcome home Joann!"

"Thank you, Ella!" Joann gave her a quick wave.

Once inside the house, Joann looked around. Everything was exactly how she left it. Nothing was out of place. This was just the way she always kept it. She walked down the hall, looking in each room as she went by, taking it all in. When she reached her bedroom, she hesitated before walking through the door.

*What will he expect of me? Will I have to perform my wifely duties? I cannot have sex after what happened to me. I cannot tell him what happened to me. I know he will hate me. He will say it was my fault.*

All of these thoughts were rolling through her unsettled mind as she stood there like a statue. John came up behind her and put his hands gently on her shoulders. Joann jumped with nervousness and fear.

He spoke kindly to her and said, "No worries, Joann. I will not ask anything of you until you are ready. I just want to be able to lay next to you in bed and know that you are there. I have missed you so much, and I love you."

Joann turned around and said, "Thank you. I needed to hear that."

The next day, John returned to work, and Joann had to go back to her life and daily duties. It would prove to be a truly tedious few weeks ahead of her, with many ups and downs, but slowly she got back into a routine. The kids were settling in, her neighbor and sister would visit constantly to see how she was doing.

Joann decided it was time to drive. She finally made her first therapy appointment. It felt good to be out and about. The kids were happy to see their grandmother, and Joann had some sense of freedom.

Life finally seemed to get back to normal for a while, and she almost felt like everything was finally turning around for her. There were some good times happening in the house, and she was eventually able to become intimate with her husband once again. Life was plugging along. Summer was in full bloom, so there were many happy family gatherings.

As summer was ending, Jon Jon was preparing to go to kindergarten. Joann had many fears about him leaving her and getting on a school bus. All the other mothers in the neighborhood were guiding her along and assured her it would be a great experience for her son.

Joann started to feel a bit of depression coming back on. It had been holding at bay for awhile, but she could feel it slowly creeping in, messing with her daily routine. The children were also starting to notice a change in her behaviors.

John just chalked it up to Joann being sad about sending her first child off to school and brushed off the many signs. Her family seemed to be on the same page with John and didn't put too much thought into it either. Now that Joann had been doing pretty good for several months, they all thought the worst was behind them. They were not checking in on her daily like they used to, and they just let life happen.

As the first day of school came closer, Joann started to struggle a bit. She became a bit edgy and short with John and the children. Joann was now getting up in the middle of the night to do extra cleaning, while everyone slept. This was something she could put her energy into, as it made her feel complete and accomplished. In the wee hours of the night, she'd be on her hands and knees scrubbing the kitchen floor with a toothbrush to make sure that she cleaned every crease

She was crying silent tears. As the wet salty fluid dripped from her cheeks, they would drop to the floor blending in with the cleaning detergent. One by one the dripping sounds became louder inside her head, and she began to scrub harder and harder with great force to try and block out the noise. All of a sudden, the toothbrush snapped—and so did Joann. She let out a ferocious scream which woke up the whole family.

The kids began to cry with fear, and John jumped out of bed thinking his family was being attacked. Like a raging bull, he came barreling down the hallway fists clenched in the air, ready to take on the world. As his feet hit the kitchen floor, he stopped dead in his tracks. The two kids were now behind him, and they all became silent just staring at her in shock.

There was John's beloved wife and mother of his children sitting on the floor in a puddle of cleaner, pulling on her hair as she's hysterically crying. She looks up at them and says, "I can't do it, do you hear me. I can't do it!" Her voice is loud and crackling.

John turns to his son and says, "Please put your sister back to bed and sit with her. Everything is alright. Mommy is just really tired."

"Ok, daddy, I will take care of Lisa."

So off Jon Jon went, taking his sister's hand. She slowly walked with him, turning back around to take a good look at her mom .

*Who is she and where did my mommy go? Will she ever come back?*

With sad eyes, Lisa turned back around and followed her brother. She knew he would always protect her.

John knelt down next to his distraught wife and held her while she cried. When she was ready, he helped her up and asked her, "Why are you doing this? I thought you were better."

She looked at him, not really knowing how to answer these questions so she responded with, "I am ok. I am just really tired. I need to go back to bed."

John put her to bed, then checked on the children who were now sleeping. He carried his son back to his own bed and went to clean up the mess.

John felt confused and angry.

*How can this be my beautiful wife all fucked up like this! What the fuck happened to her, and how am I supposed to deal with her awful behaviors?*

John pondered these thoughts, and he never made his way back to bed that night. He just sat in the darkness, smoking a cigarette with all of these intense feelings of rage, anger, and bitterness toward this situation.

*How did I get a broken wife? Why me? She needs to be fixed!*

As the morning sun was coming up, John made his way out the door to go to work. He put his thoughts and feelings aside, buried it into silence, and went about his day. Joann called him at work a few times, but he grumbled at her quickly and hung up the phone. He was very angry, and she felt completely abandoned.

This was unfortunately the new normal for John and Joann, and the children moved forward blindly with no explanations as to what was going on.

Two weeks later, John Patrick Sega started kindergarten.

John stayed home from work that day to see his son off to school for the first time. He was so proud of his little boy. John loved his children more than anything. His only son and his baby girl.

The household was filled with excitement on that morning, as the kids were loud eating their cereal and chatting about Jon Jon's big day.

Lisa looked at him and said, "I cannot believe you are leaving me. I want to go to school with you."

"I am a big boy now, and I have to go to school. My friends are waiting for me," Jon replied.

"I thought I was your friend," Lisa said with a very sad look on her face.

She was sitting there in the chair with her two ponytails swaying back and forth as she put her head down. He came over to her, and he gently put his hand on her chin, lifting up her face so she could see him. He was staring into her big blue eyes as they had a few tears in them. He kissed her on the top of her head and said, "You are more than a friend. You are my sister, and I love you. I hope you are the first one I see when I get off the bus today."

With a half-smile, Lisa agreed to be there and said, "I love you too."

This special bond between sister and brother was like no other. Jon Jon had a maturity and knowing about him that was way beyond his years. Lisa felt that from him and trusted him with every word that he said. Lisa also had a deep sense of knowing at a very young age. These two children thought on a very different level, quite different from other kids in their age group. They had deep souls.

While all of this was transpiring in the kitchen, Joann had locked herself in the bathroom and was sitting on the floor hyperventilating. As she rocked back and forth talking to herself, she felt frozen with all of her anxiety and fears claiming her body, mind, and being.

All of a sudden, she heard her husband, "Joann come on out. We have to go, it's time. What the hell are you doing in there?"

Joann jumped to her feet, turned on the water quickly, and said, "I am just washing my face. I will be right out."

John knew better, but ignored it as he made his way to the door with the kids. He just didn't want to deal with whatever was happening in there.

Out of the bathroom, she finally stepped, knowing there was no way around this. She had to face the inevitable. Her son was leaving her. She felt devastated inside, but she heard the words of her mother, "Joann be brave!"

As she faced her husband and children, she put on a smile, and they smiled too. Joann was faking it for the sake of her family, but inside she was twisting and turning as that little voice in her head was trying to reclaim his spot.

"JOANN THEY ALL REALLY HATE YOU—YOU ARE A FAILURE—LOOK AT THOSE FAKE SMILES—THEY WISH YOU WERE DEAD—MAYBE YOU SHOULD KILL YOURSELF!"

As they all made their way out of the door, Joann looked back at her empty home and whispered, "Shut up."

The Sega family walked up the street unified, as all of the other neighborhood children were gathering at the corner. Excitement filled the air, as the laughter of the kids was magnifying. If you could bottle up the energy of this big crew, you could light up New York City! Many proud parents stood chatting as the children ran around chasing each other.

Some parents were trying to round up the children for group photos documenting this momentous occasion! All of the children were dressed in their finest clothing. The little girls were in cute dresses of all colors and the boys in shirts and ties.

The bus pulled up, and it was time. The parents were kissing their kids' goodbye, and there were a few tears along the way. Overall, it was excitement, anticipation, and pride!

It was Jon Jon's turn to get on the bus. His dad hugged and kissed him, told him how extremely proud he was and that he loved him very much. His sister looked a bit lost, so Jon stuck his tongue out at her, and she laughed. Then it was his mom's turn.

Joann bent down, and he hugged her tightly. He looked at her and said, "Don't worry mommy. I am a big boy now I will be ok. I love you."

Joann said, "I know you will be, and I love you too." She ran her fingers through his thick brown hair and tickled his chin. He gave her a broad smile. Then he turned and walked away.

Jon Jon got on the bus with his friends and future class mates with a mixed amount of emotions and feelings. He was very excited but also worried about his sister. The bus pulled away, and there was no turning back now. He waved until the bus was out of sight.

Lisa jumped up and down like a wild child until he was gone. Then they turned around, said their good-byes to the neighbors, and silently walked down the street together.

Oh, that silence . . .

It became a normalcy in that house on Wildwood Terrace.

Silence and sadness.

# Chapter 9

# Fall Is Upon Us— The Great Depression

As life moved forward, Joann got into her new routine of getting up early and making sure Jon was neat as a pin and at the bus stop on time every morning.

The early morning hours were a big struggle for her, as she did not sleep most nights. The anxieties of life were riding high inside her mind as they did that dirty dance with a mixed elixir of fear, sadness, shame, and defeat. This heaviness was something that she battled every single day of her life, and the autumn season was the worst time of year for her.

As the leaves began to change and fall to the ground, so did Joann. The days become longer and heavier with shades of darkness all around her. She felt like she was in a clouded bubble trying to see through the glazed over surface.

When it came to her children, she was like a vigilant soldier marching into battle, as she pushed forward to do what was right for them. On the outside, all looked perfect in her little world of deceit.

You see, Joann was a beautiful woman who kept her home just so. There was not a thing out of place, and you could eat off of her sparkling kitchen floor, which she would scrub on her hands and knees countless times a week. Her two small children were dressed to a T, and you could always smell fresh cooking coming out of her kitchen window. The neighbor next door would frequently yell out to her, "Hey Joann, what are you cooking today? It smells great!"

Oh yes, from the outside looking in, one could become envious of this dark haired beauty who seemed to have it all. A beautiful home, a big, strong handsome husband, and two wonderful children.

As she drove around in her little gold 1965 Mustang, darting from place-to-place, people were watching and talking. Mind you, a new era was upon them. The 1960s were coming to an end, and times were changing. Joann drove her car like she felt inside. There were times that she would drive extremely slow as she was paranoid about everything, and then during her manic times, she flew like a race car driver, with her children in tow. YES, people were talking!

Sometimes some of the male neighbors would stop her husband as he was driving, and let him know that his wife had one hell of a lead foot and was a bit dangerous. John assured them that he would speak to her, and she would slow down a bit. Inside John was boiling at the fact that someone would tell him what to do about his wife, or the fact that he had to deal with it.

On one occasion, John came into the house after the neighbor up the street gave him a lecture about his wife's driving style, and he was totally annoyed. As he walked through the door, he was welcomed by his wife sitting at the table smoking a cigarette with fire in her eyes.

He said to her, "Joann, Lou just stopped me again to complain about your driving. You almost ran him over today! What the hell are you doing while I am at work?"

Joann took a big, long hard puff of her cigarette enjoying every ounce of that nicotine, closing her eyes for a moment, embracing the feeling, then she looked her husband in the eye as she exhaled a huge puff of smoke and said, "Fuck you, dickhead! Lou is a mother fucking prick who needs to mind his own fucking business." Then she spat on the floor and made a face at John, like a scolded child.

John became enraged at her, with his eyes bulging out of his head, then he started yelling. The house seemed to shake, and the children came running in from outside to see what was going on. As John ranted and raved, she sat in silence, with a perplexed look on her face.

Jon Jon and Lisa stood there with wide eyes as their father went on and on until he noticed their presence. He dashed an evil glare at Joann and looked at the kids saying, "It is ok, go back outside and play. Mommy and daddy are just having a discussion."

Jon Jon knew better as he was aware of the reality, but he did as his father said. He took his baby sister back outside. As the kids sat on the step listening to their parents scream at each other, they cried together. Jon held Lisa tight, whispering in her ear, "It will be ok, I promise."

As John and Joann's battle raged on, what they did not know was that their children were listening to every single word, as they sat in horror. They held each other tight for what seemed like an eternity until the yelling finally stopped. The house went silent until you heard the bedroom door slam shut. The kids waited a few moments and then cautiously entered the house, looking around for any sign of movement.

Joann had retreated to her bedroom, dropping to the bed as she sobbed uncontrollably. She lit up another cigarette and turned up the radio, blaring music so loud that you could hear it all the way down the street.

John went out the back door onto the deck lighting up a cigarette as well. He sat silently in the chair staring out into the yard. He was thinking about when he and Joann first met as kids. As he puffed away, he thought about how they learned how to smoke together and listened to all of the latest music of the 50s.

Then the song *Unchained Melody* came to his mind, as it was their song. As the memories came flooding back, a small tear dripped from his eye. He was losing his wife, he felt it.

*How did they get here?*

All of that love between them slowly slipping away. He shook his head in confusion, thinking to himself, *I do not know what to do.* John sat there for a very long time, as Joann's music played in the background of his mind, finally shaking him back to reality.

As sadness turned back to anger, he got up, walked back into the house storming past the children who were standing there watching him, and marched straight down the hallway as he proceeded to bang on the door with such force, he put a hole right through it. The noise was so intense that the kids went running into the living room closet and sat on the floor shaking in fear.

John's voice echoed through the house as he screamed at Joann to turn down the fucking music at once as he made his way into the bedroom. Their voices raised to the highest levels in this twisted harmony of unpleasantry, as the children shook quietly in the darkness of the closet.

It was finally over . . . John then proceeded to grab his keys as he left the house without awareness of where his children were. He was so enraged by Joann's behaviors he could not think clearly at all. He violently slammed the door as he left and jumped into his car. John sped away like a manic punching the steering wheel as he drove. He knew he had to get out of that house before he did something that he would later regret.

Jon and Lisa were profusely shaken up by what had transpired and emerged ever so slowly from the closet. Joann was walking into the kitchen when she noticed them. As she stood there for a moment with dark, scary eyes that seemed larger than life, the kids froze in terror.

Joann then unleashed all of her anger onto them as she started screaming bloody murder. The kids did not know what to do, so they just took it. Then she ordered them into their rooms to sit on their beds in silence.

"You two brats are in my closet messing it up! I will teach you both to mess up all of my stuff! Go to your rooms and do not come out until I say so!"

They scurried like little mice that were being hunted by a predator, with their little feet never hitting the floor. As they made their way past their mom, terror filled their little bodies as her unpredictable behaviors were running wild.

Jon blocked his mother's swings, protecting his little sister as he pushed her forward. When they hit the doorway of Lisa's room, he shoved her in and said, "Shut the door and do not come out until I come for you!"

Lisa nodded in fear as she shut her door and then jumped up on her bed, held her dolly as she rocked and cried.

Jon ran into his room, shut the door, and just waited and listened. It seemed like an eternity of silence. Jon waited and waited. He was a brave young man who was quite savvy for his age. He decided he needed to see what was going on, so he got off of his bed and crept to the door. He opened it up slowly, trying not to make a sound because he did not want to upset his mom. Slowly down the hallway he went. When he got to Lisa's door, he opened it and peeked in.

"Lisa, hang on. I am going to check on mommy. I will be right back for you."

"Ok Jon Jon," whimpered Lisa.

As Jon slowly made his way into the kitchen, he didn't see his mother, so he traveled into the living room. There was mommy, sitting on the couch looking out the window mumbling to herself. Jon carefully approached her and said, "Mommy are you ok?"

As she looked at her son, her heart broke. Joann had that loving look back in her eyes that were so dark and colder earlier that day.

"I am sorry Jon Jon. Mommy does not feel good."

"It is ok Mommy. I love you."

"I love you too."

He reached up and gave his mom the biggest hug ever.

She then pulled back and said to him, "How did you become such a big boy?"

He chucked and said, "because you feed me so well!" Then they both laughed.

Joann told him to go get his sister, and she would make them dinner. He did as he was told, and Jon and Lisa sat quietly watching TV until dinner was ready. The three of them ate in silence together. There were so many silent emotions flying around the table that night—fear, sadness, anger, shame, confusion, and guilt. That is what was served up at this table of disaster, along with spaghetti and meatballs.

Joann mustered up every ounce of strength as she cleaned up the mess, got her children bathed and ready for bed. She read to them out of Lisa's book of nursery rhymes and then kissed them both on the forehead, tucking them in for the night, promising that tomorrow would be a better day.

The children took comfort in those empty words, hoping it would be true. As they listened to their mom make her way back down the hallway, it was not a lullaby that cradled them to sleep, but the sound of Joann's tears.

As all of this transpired, John was sitting on the beach with a six pack of cold beer, listening to the waves crash against the rocks. He pondered for a very long time as the sun set, and the moon rose. Staring at the stars, he prayed. He asked God to help his wife and deteriorating family. When the last can was empty, he finally got back up and made his way slowly home, wondering what he would find when he got there.

Then his mind shifted to the children, and he realized in all of that chaos he never saw them when he walked out. Now anxiety and fear washed over him, as he drove a bit faster racing to get back home, with every horrible thought going through his head.

*What an idiot I am! I am an awful father leaving my children like that! What if she harmed them, or they are lost in the woods behind our house alone and scared! What have I done?*

John pulled up in front of the house, panicked as he ran toward the steps. He lept up the steps and made his way through the unlocked door. There was a pit in his stomach as sweat was beading on his brow. As he came across the threshold, he stopped. There was silence—complete silence. He looked over into the living room, and there was Joann sound asleep on the couch. John made his way down the hallway to check on his children.

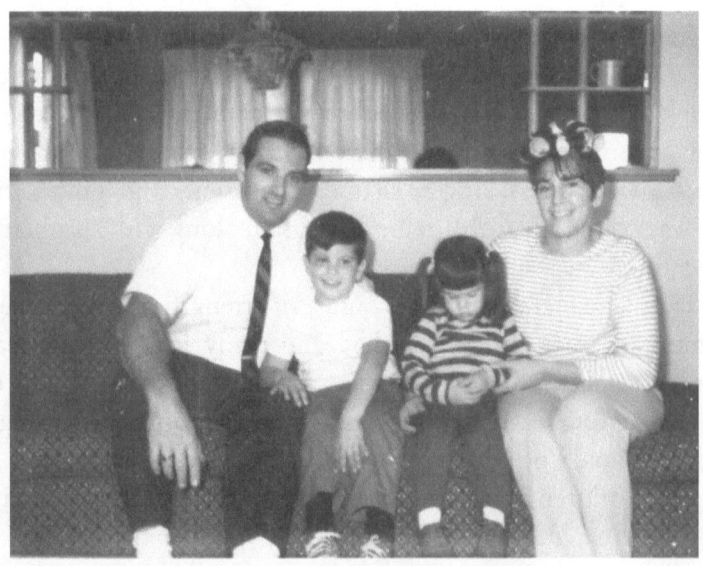

*Family 1968*

Lisa and Jon were both tucked away in their beds safe and sound. John let out a big sigh of relief, as guilt rushed through his entire body. He then made his way back to his wife. He gently leaned down and kissed her forehead and covered her with a blanket. John sat down in the chair next to the couch and watched his beautiful wife sleep so peacefully. There were so many thoughts going through his head, and all he wanted to do was save his wife—but he had no idea how.

He whispered to himself, "I am losing my family. What am I supposed to do?"

Big Bad John felt helpless for the first time in his entire life.

# Chapter 10

# When Leukemia Strikes

John Patrick Sega was a beautiful little boy with dark brown hair, and big chocolate brown eyes. His skin had a hint of that deep olive glow of many Italian children. As the oldest child of the family, he was a natural born leader to his younger sister Lisa.

Jon Jon, as he was affectionally called throughout his short life, was how most people referred to him. He had a stocky strong build, and he loved his pasta and meatballs. Jon had a laugh that would put an instant smile on your face, as his expressions were larger than life when he spoke.

The best things about little Jon were that he had a kind heart and deep compassion for others, even at such a young tender age of seven. He made friends where ever he went, and in school he was a leader in the classroom. Jon also loved sports, with baseball being his absolute favorite.

He was the pride and joy of his young family, and he was put on a pedestal so to speak. The first born child to John and Joann, a beautiful healthy baby boy, how could one not be proud! Everyone in the family always doted over him, and he was spoiled (in a good way).

As he grew from being a beautiful baby into a little boy, he had such wonder about everything, especially nature. Jon Jon was a busy little boy with so much energy, and his imagination ran "to infinity and beyond." If he was not outside playing with his Tonka Trucks, or running around with his friends, you could find him in his room playing with his castle filled with knights, or racing his Hot Wheel cars. There was always a great adventure, and he loved taking his little sister along for the ride.

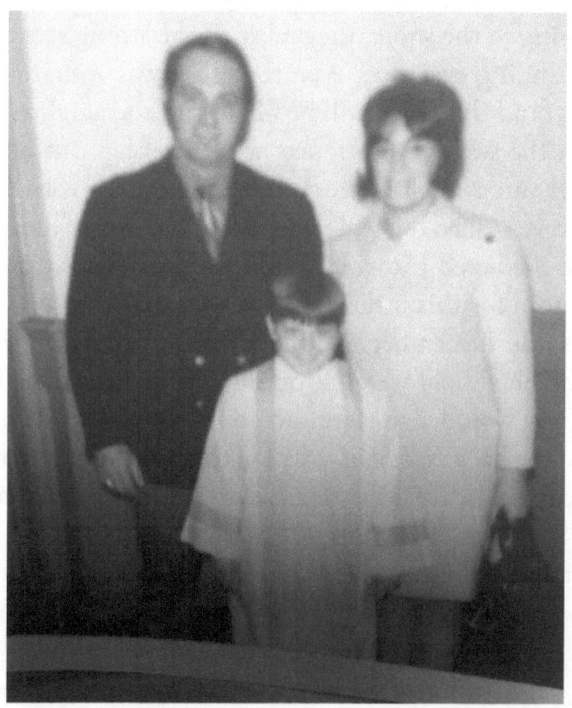

*Jon Jon First Communion*

Jon Jon had a special place in his heart for Lisa, and he spent a lot of time with her. He felt a natural protective way about her and knew he had to keep her safe. When the household would become unstable, his immediate thoughts went to her, and he would go into protection mode. Lisa could always count on him to shield her from any storm that came crashing down on this beautiful home on Wildwood Terrace.

Could anyone every look at Jon Jon and think—
He is sick?
NO . . .

**Christmas Eve 1970—**

As the fall air turned into the winter chill, you could feel the essence of snow all around New England. This beautiful little town in West Haven by the shore was preparing for the holiday season. The salt water turned cold and a bit dark, but when the beautiful waves came crashing to the shore, they released the strong scent of salt into the air reminding everyone, even though it was winter, the sun will shine again, and the beach will be filled with the laughter of children running in the waves. Vacationers will travel far and wide to enjoy the summer sun as their bodies bronze and glisten with exotic oils.

The waves called out as a reminder of renewal of life, but nobody could have predicted those dark cold waters were a warning sign of what lay ahead for this little family by the sea.

It was mid-December, and the town lit up like a huge Christmas village. The neighbors were all outside decorating their homes and yards. People would drive around from street to street with their children in the back seats excitedly looking out the window admiring all the decorations. It was a magical time of year, and everyone was celebrating!

Joann loved this time of year; it was her favorite. She never felt so alive as she did in the month of December. Her home was decorated inside and out. It looked like one of the houses in *Better Homes and Gardens*. Joann made sure everything was perfect. Every ornament had a place, the manger was done just so, and the lights outside shined ever so brightly. The smells that came from the kitchen were heavenly, as she baked daily right until Christmas Eve.

The children were so excited as the days came closer. They could hardly contain themselves, as they jumped up and down singing Christmas carols and sitting under the tree admiring the decorations. The smell of pine filled the room, as the broad tree stood before the picture window, like a beacon of light and hope. During this time of year, everyone in the household seemed happy, like they were living in a bubble of protection. They all embraced the magic.

John and Joann took the kids to see Santa and went out for long drives admiring all the neighborhoods. They would come back home and have hot cocoa with marshmallows and watch all the Christmas shows on television. Looking at this family, one would never think that they had so much dysfunction and sadness in their home. From the outside looking in, many thought it was a perfect life filled with love and happiness. If the walls could talk . . .

Finally, Christmas Eve arrived, and the day seemed so long for the children as they were waiting impatiently to start the festivities. The stockings were hung, the presents were wrapped, and the lists for Santa delivered.

Jon Jon woke up that day not feeling so well, but it did not stop him from feeling excitement. Children as so resilient even when they are feeling under the weather. Joann did notice that he wasn't acting himself but brushed it off as possibly being a cold.

John went to work but assured Joann he would be home early so they could all travel to his parent's house for a big Christmas Eve and the Feast of the Seven Fishes! It was a huge tradition, and the house would be bursting at the seams, with family and friends enjoying wine, eating fantastic food with an endless display of desserts. The children would run rampant through the house, with such high sounds of laughter the roof might pop off. Yes, a magical time for all.

Nothing like strong family traditions to end the year!

Joann was busy in the kitchen finishing up her last-minute baking, when Jon Jon entered the room.

"Mommy, I have a bad headache."

Joann turned around a bit annoyed at being disturbed, but when she saw the look on his face and how pale he was, she felt a bit concerned.

"Jon Jon, you have a headache, does anything else hurt?"

"No, just my head, and I feel this pain in my chest."

Joann went right to the medicine cabinet, pulled out the St. Joseph baby aspirin, and gave him four little pink chewable tablets. Jon Jon seemed happy to take them because as kids growing up in that era of the 1970s, these little pills seemed more like candy then medicine. Joann walked him over to the couch and took his temperature.

At this moment, Lisa came around the corner to see what was going on and saw her brother laying on the couch.

"What is wrong Mommy?"

"Oh, your brother has a headache and a low fever. Lay here Jon Jon. I'll go get a cool cloth for your head."

As Joann rushed past Lisa ignoring the distressed look on her little face, she walked over to her brother and asked, "Are you ok? You cannot be sick. Santa is coming tonight."

"I know, I know. I am fine. I have this headache, and my chest hurts."

Joann came back into the living room, placed a cool white cloth on his forehead, and sent Lisa back into the other room so he could rest.

"Lisa, go back in your room and play with your dolls; your brother needs to nap right now."

"OK Mommy."

As Lisa looked up at her mom, she looked so angry. Lisa felt a bit uneasy as she slowly walked away, drooping her head down, and shuffling her feet.

Joann went back into the kitchen to finish up everything before her husband came home. Jon Jon fell asleep for a long time. Joann didn't even realize how long because she was so pre-occupied, until her husband came through the door. As she looked up at him, she was reminded of her son. As John came walking towards her, that is when she stated that their son was not feeling well.

John went right over to him, and Jon Jon opened his eyes.

"Hey buddy what is going on"?

"Hi Daddy, I have a headache."

"Oh, you cannot have a headache today. It's Christmas Eve, and we have a party to go to."

"Yes daddy, I want to go."

John looked at his son for a moment and could see that his coloring was off. Jon Jon gave him a half smile.

Suddenly Lisa came bursting into the room and jumped on her daddy's back so excited to see him.

"Hey there is my little girl. Are you all ready for Santa?"

"Yes, daddy yes!" Lisa shouted as she jumped up and down.

John got up, and she took him by the hand to show him all of the presents under the tree.

"Mommy wrapped today!" Lisa squealed with excitement.

"I see that! Do you think there is a present under there for your daddy?"

"Yes, yes! The big blue one daddy! We shopped together."

Jon Jon managed to get up and wanted to join in on the action, trying not to show them that he really was not feeling well.

"That's my boy, you are up and moving. I knew you were fine. Your mom likes to overreact at times," John stated.

Joann shot him a look of pure annoyance.

"Ok, ok," said Joann. "Let's get this show on the road."

She sent the children off to brush their teeth and get changed into their special Christmas attire. John took a quick shower, and Joann packed up all of the food and gifts. The children came back out, and she brushed their hair and made them look just so.

Jon Jon was hiding the fact that he felt so sick, but he did not want to miss a thing so when his mother pulled him close.

"Jon Jon, are you sure you feel better?"

He answered that he was fine. He looked so handsome in his blue dress pants, grey shirt with a holiday tie. The brown loafers on his feet finished the look. Joann admired her boy, thinking about how handsome he was, but she felt that the usual sparkles in his eyes were missing.

She then shifted her attention to Lisa.

Now, Lisa was in the finest little dress from Macy's. It was green velvet with ruffles. The color matched the stripes in Jon Jon's tie. She had trouble putting on her tights, so her mom fixed them and helped her buckle her patent leather shoes. Joann brushed out her long hair, then pulled some back on top, and pinned a beautiful bow in it to finish the look.

John came into the room, and they both admired how beautiful their children were. They smiled at each other, feeling a sense of pride and accomplishment for getting this far together. They doted on the kids for a few moments.

Joann instructed John to take some pictures in front of the Christmas tree while she got changed.

When Joann came waltzing back into the room with her floral dress, she looked stunning. John commented on how beautiful she looked and gave her a kiss under the mistletoe. The kids giggled at their parents, and off they went.

It was time for Christmas Eve to begin.

## The Collapse . . .

As they pulled up to the house, there were already family members gathering. The front porch light shined brightly, and the kids could see family in the screened in porch, waiting to enter with many gifts in hand.

Lisa was bouncing up and down in the backseat squealing with the sight before her eyes.

"Ok, ok, calm down, Lisa. You're shaking the car!" stated her Dad, as he was laughing.

John looked back at his son sitting there extremely quiet, next to his sister. He paused for a moment, and then said, "Let's get out and go have some fun!" Everyone exited the vehicle, as John opened the trunk to take out all of the food and presents. Jon Jon grabbed his mother's hand as they walk up the side walk with Lisa running up ahead.

As they made their way inside, it was a full house and the energy level was through the roof. Lisa dropped her coat on the floor and took off running. Joann picked it up as they entered the house. She knelt down and once again asked her son if he was ok, this time really staring into his eyes. He insisted he was fine, but just feeling very tired. Joann took his coat from him and sent him off to see his cousins.

John came in behind her, and she whispered to him, "I don't think Jon Jon is ok. Please keep an eye on him."

"I will," John said looking uptight.

John then made his way through the crowd carrying the food as he hugged and kissed people along the way. His mom and dad were busy in the kitchen preparing food. He put down his items and kissed his mom on the cheek.

"Merry Christmas Mom," he said.

She smiled at him and said, "Let's get some of this food out on the table. We need some more room in here."

John turned his attention to his dad. John loved his dad beyond the moon and back. His father was his true hero. He walked over, picked his dad up, and gave him a bear hug.

"Put me down, you crazy fool!" his dad said with a huge smile on his face.

John kissed him on top of his balding head and said, "Merry Christmas Dad!" He put him down and then did what his mother asked of him, because she was looking at him with a look of contempt! John and his father both started laughing.

As the family gathered around the table, the wine was being poured, and the kids were settling in at the kids' table with sodas in hand.

They said a Christmas blessing and all dug into the magnificent feast. There was so much laughter, love, and magic flying all over the room that evening. It was a perfect Christmas Eve for all.

When dinner was over, the women got up from the table and started to clear all the dishes, as the men sat chatting about life. It was so classic for the sign of the times.

The men were smoking cigarettes, and the room filled with ringlets of smoke. The women were in the kitchen organizing the mess, as the children ran from room to room chanting and yelling about opening presents. They were all so excited. Jon Jon, on the other hand, was sitting on the couch looking quite lethargic.

John noticed his son's absence from the sea of children flowing through the dining room and became concerned. He got up and went into the living room. He found Jon sitting on the couch.

"Hey buddy, what's up? You're not playing with the other kids."

Jon looked at his dad and said, "I feel dizzy. I need to get up."

John grabbed him by the hand, and as Jon Jon stood up, his eyes rolled back in his head and he dropped to the floor shaking, then passed out cold!

John let out a huge yell that could have exploded a building, and everyone came running! Joann broke through the crowd of people to see her son, lying on the ground shaking as John was holding him tightly screaming his name!

Lisa could hear the screaming and crawled under the table and through the legs of everyone to get to her brother! Lisa was horrified at the sight before her, as Joann was hysterically crying!

Everyone was frozen in this moment of time, shocked at the sight before them. This was supposed to be a celebration, a holy night of the angels with excited children waiting for Santa to arrive.

How can this be?

"Jon Jon, it is daddy can you hear me? Please answer me!" John repeated himself over and over again.

Joann was sobbing uncontrollably with her sister-in-law by her side trying to hold her back. Little Lisa stood in horror not understanding what she was seeing, so terrified that she wet herself, as tears streamed down her face.

Jon finally opened his eyes and whispered, "Daddy."

John held his son up to his chest so tightly saying, "Son please don't leave us!"

"I won't daddy, but I feel really bad."

"It will be alright. We are going to go see the doctor, and he will make it all better. I promise."

Jon looked into his dad's eyes and everything was blurry. "I can't see you daddy. It's dark."

John looked at Joann and said, "We are going to the hospital right now. Pull yourself together, do you hear me!" John's tone was gruff and cold.

Joann looked at him with eyes as wide as a deer in the headlights, and she just nodded her head.

John picked his son up off the floor and told him they were going to the hospital and everything would be ok. John's mother wrapped a knitted blanket around him, as Joann grabbed her purse.

As they were rushing out the door, Lisa let out a big scream, "NO NO, don't take my brother away from me!"

Her grandfather came over and swooped her up, and held her tight as tears began to flow.

Just like that they were gone, and everyone stood there in silence, which seemed like forever.

How did such a perfect family gathering, turn into such a nightmare with the flick of a switch? It was so over-whelming as many were crying. Some were just sitting there, shaking their heads as others made their way out on the back porch to get some fresh air and smoke.

Lisa held onto her grandfather tightly, and then pulled back looking him in the eyes and said, "I peed my pants. I am all wet."

"It is alright," her grandfather said. "Let's get you to grandma so she can change you."

He put her down, and they went into the kitchen. He handed her off to his wife as he was so overwhelmed with emotions. He wept in the corner of the kitchen by himself.

Theresa brought Lisa in the bathroom and helped her get cleaned up. She was a strong woman who rarely showed emotions.

Lisa looked up at her and said, "Will my brother be ok grandma?"

Theresa looked down at her distraught granddaughter and simply said, "He will be fine. Let's go, I have to clean up that kitchen."

Lisa put her head down, hurt, confused, and a bit angry for reasons that she could not even understand, but she did as her grandmother told her and got changed.

As they left the bathroom, not another word was said, and Lisa made her way out into the sea of family, feeling so desperately alone and completely invisible. She made her way over to the couch and curled up in the exact spot that her brother was sitting not so long ago. She could still smell him, as a few tears rolled down her little pink cheeks. She took in some air and then shook silently until she fell asleep. All the noise in the house cradled her as the chaos and trauma was just too much for her to handle. Her grandfather came over and covered her with a blanket.

**The Hospital Run . . .**

The drive to the hospital was silent. Joann sat in the backseat holding her son tight as he let out a few whimpers. John was fixated on the path that he needed to take to get them there as quickly as possible. Sweat was beading from his brow, as his hands were frozen tight on the wheel. Many thoughts were racing through his head, but he had to remain focused on getting them there in one piece.

When he pulled up in front of the emergency room, he instructed Joann to stay in the car with their son. John burst through the door with such force, everyone stopped and took notice. He ran to the desk in a panic.

"Please help us. My son passed out and is very sick! He is out in the car with my wife, hurry up! Now, let's go Now!" He was screaming so loud it felt like the building was shaking.

The nurses ran out immediately bringing a wheelchair. As they pulled him out from Joann's arms, she was crying, "My son, my son, please help him!"

John helped her out of the car, and they followed the team of nurses inside. They were ushered immediately in the back, as the doctors were called in. So many things were happening at one time, and little Jon was terrified.

"I can't breathe! I can't breathe," he kept on repeating.

John and Joann stood there feeling helpless as the doctor worked on their son. The doctor ordered a battery of tests and had the nurse escort them to the waiting room. They did not want to leave their son but were forced out gently by the staff.

It seemed like eternity as they waited. Joann sat motionless in a chair looking like a mannequin with a blank expression on her face. John paced uncontrollably back and forth with such rage and anger that the nurses were afraid to approach him.

Finally, after what seemed like days instead of hours, the doctor emerged. As he walked in, he had a look on his face that John feared.

"Please sit down, I have the results of your son's tests."

John snapped back at him, "Where is my son? I need to see him now!"

"We will go back in a few moments. I am sorry for all of this waiting, but we wanted to make sure of the results." The doctor put his head down for a moment, took in a deep breath and said, "Your son has Leukemia and a tumor in his chest."

Joann starting quietly sobbing, "Noooo, nooo, noooo, this can't be, nooooo!"

John felt the blow of these fatal words as he took it all in, glancing over at his distraught wife, and back at the doctor.

"What are you saying to us? Is he going to die?"

With an apologetic look, the doctor started to explain what treatments would be available to them. He talked about chemotherapy and radiation. Many medications would be needed to try and shrink the tumor in his chest. It must be done immediately, as the tumor was putting pressure on Jon Jon's lungs. That was why he was having trouble breathing.

John was silent as he reached for Joann's hand. She pushed it away, as she continued to cry. He felt destroyed inside, thinking,

*First my wife and now my son! Are you fucking kidding me?* He felt so incredibly alone in that moment. As his heart was breaking, he simply said, "I need to see my child now."

The doctor brought them in to see Jon Jon. He was laying there looking so weak. John went over and touched the top of his head gently.

"Hey buddy, it's me, daddy."

Jon opened his eyes and gave him a half smile, "Daddy, I want to go home. Santa won't come unless I am in my bed."

With a simple tear in his eye, John said, "It's ok son. Santa will come to you. I promise."

"Mommy, Mommy, are you here?"

Joann mustered up the courage to walk forward to be there for her son.

She was broken inside as she looked at her beautiful child seeming so weak and helpless. She smiled and said, "I am right here always."

As both parents stood at each side of his bed, Jon smiled and said, "I love you both so much."

Joann kissed his forehead and said, "We love you too."

The meaning of Christmas was forever changed.

This incredible little family was being picked apart slowly by circumstance and time. They were ripped apart by so many traumatic events that were bigger than all of them. They could not fight the fate that lay ahead for each one of them. All four of them traveled down a different road of, loss, pain, suffering, dysfunction and abuse.

**The Unspoken Truth—A story to be told many years later.**

### John Patrick Sega—His Journey

Jon Jon was a special little boy with many gifts to offer anyone who was in his presence. There was an essence about him that could only be described as heavenly. He was a son, brother, grandchild, nephew, cousin, and friend. He fought gallantly for two years with this awful disease. Never wavering in his good nature, humor and strength. His kindness and compassion stood strong.

Through all of the chemotherapy and radiation treatments, he remained determined and loving. It was as if he knew what was to come but chose to live in the moments as they came to fruition. He did not want to miss a thing!

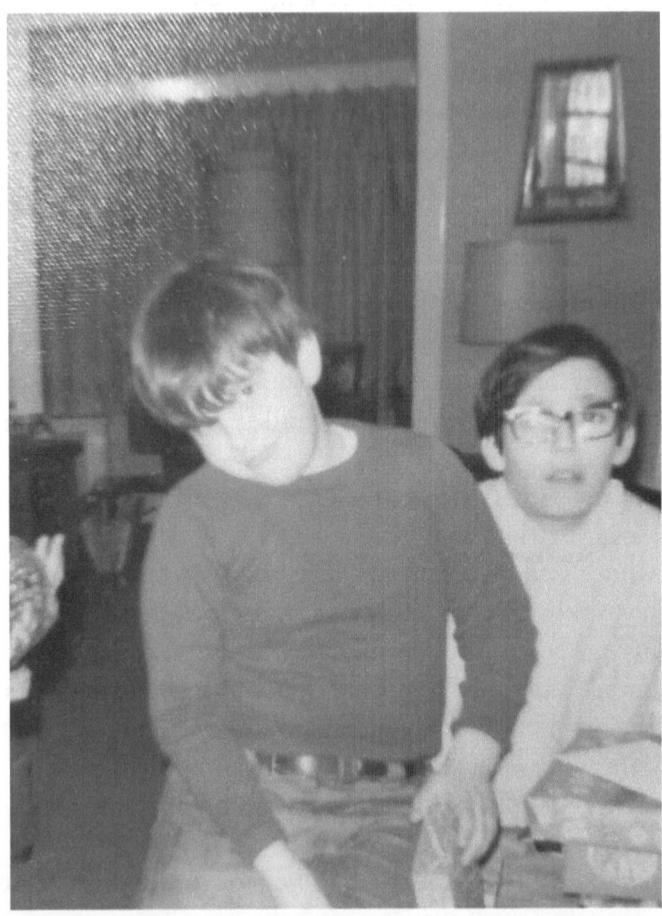

*March 1972 Jon Jon 9th birthday he passed away April 22, 1972*

Just before it was his time to return home to the Lord, he had a special conversation with his sister Lisa about the visit he had with the angels. They told him he would be called home soon. Lisa asked if the angels would come to visit her next and stated that she did not want him to leave her. She also wanted to know if they could both get wings so they could fly like the birds in the sky.

As they laughed and cried together, they solidified a bond that could never be broken in life or death.

On April 22, 1972, John passed away at the tender age of just nine years old.

His family was left devastated, and that is when the true downward spiral began.

Big John always said that he lost his son and wife on that dreadful day— He was correct.

**Stepping Forward**

The days and weeks after Jon Jon's death proved to be challenging for all. The struggle to just get up every day and try to regain control of life, hoping to bring things back to some kind of normal!

*Normal—what does that mean after the passing of a child?*

Life will never be normal again, and how do you recover from such a devastating blow? No parent should ever have to bury their child. It is not normal or natural.

It was only one day after the funeral that John decided to return to work, leaving Joann in a puddle of grief. She was riddled with depression and mania all in one. She also had the responsibility of a small child to care for.

Lisa was also feeling lost and vulnerable at this time. She was not allowed to go to the wake or funeral, which left her in such a state of confusion about what really happened to her brother.

*Why did he have to go away, and why couldn't she say good-bye?* There were no other explanations, only the words of her father.

"Your brother is gone. He is now in heaven with the angels."

Those words continued to roll over and over in her mind as she sat on the floor in her bedroom playing with her dolls. The echo was so painful, and the imagery was like a moving picture show inside her head.

"Your brother is no longer with us anymore; he went to heaven to be with the angels." These were the words of her distraught father on the day of Jon's passing.

As he was sitting on the floor with his head in her lap sobbing uncontrollably, Lisa stroked his hair, not knowing what else to do, she leaned over and whispered in his ear, "It is ok daddy. You still have me."

The thoughts and images continued to roll over and over inside her brain as the echo became louder. These silent emotions were filling her soul with sadness and anger.

She yelled out loud in distress, "I hate the angels!" She then threw her baby doll across the room. She ran over to her bed and jumped up onto it, grabbing her teddy bear, squeezing it tightly and began to cry.

*Jon Jon, please come home! I miss you. Where are you? Is it dark there? You are afraid of the dark, and I cannot help you. Please angels, please send him back home. I need him!"*

As the tears continued to flow, Lisa could hear something coming from the other room. She sat up straight on her bed half scared and half excited.

There were noises coming from Jon Jon's room.

"They brought him back!" Lisa whispered to her bear. She jumped off the bed and ran down the hall wanting to see him standing there with his broad smile and open arms! Instead, she was met with an image that would stay in her mind for years to come.

As Lisa stood in the doorway of her brother's room, she stopped dead in her tracks. Standing there holding her pink bear, she was devasted. Instead of being greeted by her brother, she was met with her sick mother laying on his bed curled up in a ball gripping his pillow ever so tightly. She was rocking back and forth crying. She had her back to the door so she never saw Lisa standing there. Lisa watched her mother silently, taking in the image of her brother's empty room and her destroyed mom. She was scared. As her mom whimpered profusely, silent tears rolled down her face.

Joann was talking out loud cursing God for taking her only son, and saying, "I have nothing left."

Those words cut Lisa like a knife, damaging her heart forever. As she continued to stand there, her thoughts shifted to her father. She wanted her daddy, but he was not there — and she felt so alone.

Walking slowly back to her room with her head hanging down, Lisa felt like nobody wanted her or loved her anymore.

*Now that Jon Jon is gone, I am alone . . . My mom doesn't want me. and my dad isn't here. I am a nobody.*

She felt invisible.

These are the thoughts of a traumatized six-year-old left alone with a grieving mother who also battled mental illness.

The more Joann needed her husband to be by her side and understand her internal struggles, the more he ran away. He immersed himself in his, and after work activities. The pain of his loss was too much to bear. He chose to hide it all as he continued to run.

The death of a child does many things to a family, and for us, it truly was the proverbial bomb that destroyed everything.

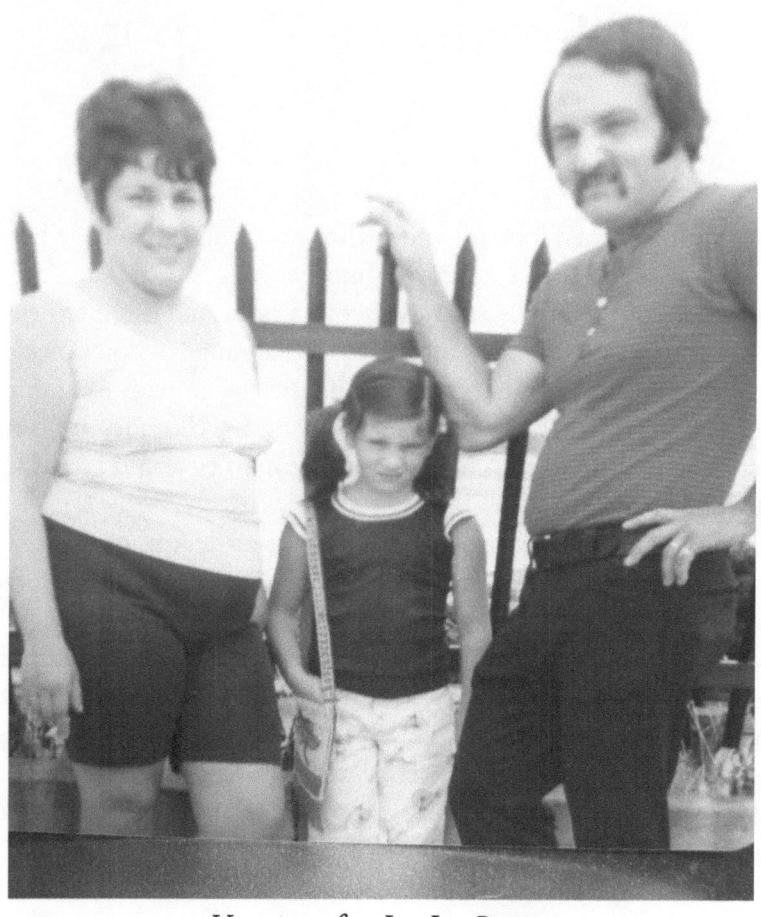

*Vacation after Jon Jon Passing*

# Chapter 11

# The Stories of My Youth

Time moved forward and Joann was trying to navigate herself through life as a grieving mother of a "dead child," as she would so boldly state to anyone who would listen to her.

Joann was on a roller coaster of a wide range of emotions, and she began to develop different personalities to go with each one of them. Unfortunately, Lisa was taken along for the ride, and was a first-hand witness to the changes that her mother would go through on a daily basis.

As Joann cycled through deep times of depression and rapid mania, Lisa was her main victim to countless bizzare moments, dangerous episodes, and vulgar behaviors. You never knew what Joann you would get next, and Lisa was always trying to figure her out as she was pummeled over, and over again with another view of mental illness at its worst.

Trying to keep up the pace of a sick parent proved to be quite difficult, disturbing and left a long string of damage to this young child.

*How does a young girl survive the trauma?*

**Valentines Day**

I watched my mother struggle daily, and though it was hard for me, even at the tender young age of ten, I wanted to help my mother. I wanted her to smile and be happy. I wanted to fix her. I thought about it all the time as I analyzed her. As I studied her, I always thought: what could I do to make it all better.

So, in the mind of a ten-year-old, what sounded perfect? The answer was chocolate!

It was Valentine's Day, and as usual, we were home alone. My mother was sitting on the couch smoking and crying (her usual MO), and I was going about my daily business.

Joann had her music playing on the stereo. Of course, it was always sad songs when she was in this state of mind. Her depression had hit hard with the cold winter winds blowing, and she couldn't seem to move. The lead weights of mental illness holding her down, relentlessly bashing away at her sanity.

I announced that I wanted to go out and take a walk. My mother barely looked over at me as she didn't seem to comprehend or care what I was actually saying. As she continued on crying and singing, I made my way out into the cold. I was all bundled up and prepared for my adventure.

I walked down to the local pharmacy, which was quite a distance from our house. By the time I got there, I was frozen solid, but I was on a mission. As I browsed through the store warming up, I found exactly what I was looking for. It was the biggest box of Russel Stover candies in the store. It was heart shaped with red and white lace on the cover. You could smell the delicious scent of chocolate right through the box. I picked it up, not even noticing the expensive price tag, and with a sense of accomplishment, I proceeded to pick out a card to go with it.

As I made my way to the counter, I put my items up on the shelf. Of course, I added in some M & Ms for myself. I was smiling brightly as the pharmacist came to the counter.

"Well, hello there. What do we have here?" the pharmacist asked.

"I have a gift for my mom. She is sick, and I wanted to make her happy," Lisa replied.

"What a kind thing to do," the man smiled. As he rang me up, the total came to over thirty dollars.

I looked at him feeling a bit uptight, and a little embarrassed as I said, "I do not have any money. Please put it on my credit."

The pharmacist asked me the family name and then said, "Are you sure this is ok with your parents?"

"Of course it is, because it will be the one thing that will make my mom feel better today."

The pharmacist agreed and charged it to our account. Just like that I had my solution in hand. I thanked him and made my way back out the door, preparing for the long trek home.

When I finally made it back, my mom was still in the exact same spot that I left her in. I took off my coat and hat, shook my long hair, as it had started to snow, and made my way over to the couch.

As I looked around at our living room, it was so pretty. The big picture window in the front with the blue and white floral couch under it. The curtains were tailored to match the fabric on the couch. The blue shag rug screamed the sign of the times, but everything was perfect, just like in the magazines.

Sometimes I would sit in this room, and I would imagine us being that family in the magazine where everything was beautiful and happy. Unfortunately, the reality was far from the truth.

The thoughts of a child shifting to fantasy to protect the heart—so classic.

"Mommy, I have something for you," Lisa said softly.

Joann looked up at her daughter with soak-filled eyes, black mascara running down her face like a muddy stream.

"What do you have for me?" Joann asked sadly.

"Happy Valentine's Day! I know chocolates are your favorite," Lisa said.

Joann held them in her hand for a moment and then gave her daughter a big smile. She leaned over and kissed her on the head.

"Thank you so much. This makes me happy! I love you my beautiful blue-eyed angel from heaven!" Joann seemed genuinely happy in the moment. I felt such pride as my mom gave me praise.

This was only to last for a short moment, but I learned throughout my young life that those moments were very important for the both of us.

Note: A Sign of the time of the Seventies.

Lisa at the age of only ten years old, went into a local store, and asked to charge items to the family's account. Without hesitation the pharmacist completed this transaction.

The downside to this was when John got the bill, he was furious at Lisa for spending so much money, and she got in major trouble. John went to the pharmacy with that bill in hand and gave the pharmacist a piece of his mind with Lisa by his side.

This was a one-time deal!

## The Tag Sale

John and his brother-in-law were pickers in their spare time on the weekends. They loved cleaning out old houses, hotels, and businesses. Most of the items would end up in John's basement, and the rest of the items went to scrap for cash. This was a great way to earn extra money, and they both loved antiquing.

On Sundays they would set up shop at the local flea market in New Haven and sell all of their fabulous treasures!

During the week of course, John was always busy working, and many times he would work late into the evening. He had no idea what would transpire in his home during the day when Lisa was left home alone with her mom.

One day Lisa said to her mom, "I am going to have a tag sale in the driveway and sell some of my things."

Joann was oblivious to so much at this point, she just nodded, shooing her away. She then went about the robotic motions of her daily routine.

Lisa was quite excited as she took some of her things from her playroom downstairs to the basement. As Lisa hit the bottom steps to the basement, she looked around at all of the items that her dad had stored away. She was intrigued by all the interesting pieces of furniture, and glass figurines stacked everywhere. Her mind raced with excitement as she imagined the stories attached to these precious gems. She had the same love of antiques just like her dad.

As she ran her hand over the items, she had a grand idea.

Lisa ran back upstairs and made a sign.

"Big Tag Sale in the Garage. Come IN!"

As she opened the garage door, the fresh air hit her. It was a warm sunny day, and the thought of selling these items to get money was enticing. Lisa happily hung up two signs. One at the end of the road with her address and one in front of the house.

She took a table and set it up outside in the driveway, with the garage door wide open. She pulled up one of the old antique chairs and sat down to wait. Slowly people came on by, and if they didn't like what was on the table, she guided them into the garage. Lisa chatted endlessly about these wonderful items, and people were listening.

There was an old antique cash register sitting there on the table, and as people began to buy different items, she stored the money in there. She was feeling so proud of herself for thinking about this, and people continued to come.

Some of the neighborhood kids stopped in and happily bought some of her dolls and games. As the day went on, it became quiet until this red car pulled up. A man stepped out of the car and approached Lisa.

"Hello there pretty girl, how are you today?" he asked.

"I am fine sir. How are you?"

"I am great now that I see you, and all this fine stuff that you are selling."

Lisa felt slightly awkward because this man was staring directly into her eyes as he spoke to her. She felt his glances like they were going through her. It made her feel uncomfortable.

"Where are your parents? Do they let you sell this stuff all by yourself? How old are you?" the man asked her.

*So many questions,* Lisa thought, but brushed the feelings aside as she answered.

"My dad is working, and my mom is in the house cleaning. They always let me do this, and it is my job. I am almost eleven-years-old you know, so I know what I am doing," Lisa said with confidence.

It seemed like she was trying to convince herself more than him, and he took great notice to it. The man looked at her with a sheepish smile and said, "Oh I bet you are a confident girl, aren't you?"

As he started to walk toward her, she backed away a bit. He stopped at the old chest of drawers and ran his hand across it.

"Oh this is smooth, like a baby's naked bottom, mmmmhhhh!"

Lisa didn't know what to say as she felt totally uncomfortable because his mood and tone of voice changed. Then he made a bit of a groan as he adjusted his private area.

Lisa piped up quickly, "Would you like to buy it, it's cheap? You can have it for thirty dollars."

"Oh, I can, really?" said the man. "That would be nice."

"Ok then, would you like to take it now?"

The man quickly replied, "Oh yes I would love to take it, that is for sure."

Lisa realized that this man was not talking about the furniture and quickly moved toward the open garage door to get outside. He quickly followed her as she made her way into the sunlight.

The look in his eyes was alarming, and Lisa didn't know what to do, so she started to talk really fast blurting out anything that she could to keep the conversation moving.

"Ok, I will go and get my truck and come back for this. Will you be waiting for me?" the man said,

"Yes, I will be here."

As the man walked toward his vehicle, he turned and said with a a devilish grin, "Now don't sell that to anyone else because its mine."

"OK I won't," Lisa replied.

When the man drove off, Lisa breathed a sigh of relief. She ran back into the garage, closing and locking the door.

She ran up the stairs into the house and directly to her room. Her mother was on the bed laying down listening to her music so loudly that she didn't even take notice to daughter's panicking footsteps.

A little while later, John came home and called Lisa out into the kitchen. As Lisa came out, her mom was sitting at the table looking very annoyed. John was holding up the sign that was posted at the top of the road.

"Lisa did you have a tag sale today?"

Lisa shot a quick look at her mom and realized she was on her own.

"Yes, dad, I did, and I did a great job too. People really loved all of your stuff in the basement. I felt just like you down at the flea market. I am just like you, dad, I am good at selling things too." Lisa was really trying to state her case.

John became furious and started yelling at her.

"Did you let strangers into the house? Did you sell my stuff? What is wrong with you! That is dangerous! Joann, why did you let her do that? Are you fucking stupid?" He was now completely angry at the both of them.

Lisa began to cry and ran to her room slamming the door.

Joann looked at him with contempt in her eyes and simply said, "Go fuck yourself." Then proceeded to spit on the floor.

This was her go to response for everything. She then lit up her cigarette and told him to go talk to someone who cared.

John walked away quickly before he did something that he didn't want to do. He was raging as he marched down the stairs to the basement slamming the door so loud that the walls shook.

As he was in the garage taking inventory of all the items Lisa sold, he heard a knocking at the door. He opened the garage door to see a big man standing there.

There was a blue van parked out front. The man looked completely startled to see John, as he was expecting to see Lisa instead.

Before the man could get a word out, John said to him, "What the fuck do you want?"

The man stuttered a bit and said he was there for the dresser. He then stupidly asked for the little girl.

John blew a gasket and grabbed this man by the shirt.

"Stay away from my house and stay away from my daughter. Do you hear me ? I will kill you! The tag sale is over, and I suggest you leave now!" He continued to hold onto this man's shirt.

Lisa heard the yelling and peeked out the window. She saw the man with the blue van, as her dad was screaming and reading him the riot act! She was terrified and hid in the closet.

She heard her dad yelling more and more, and then she heard a door slam as the vehicle went speeding off. The garage door slammed shut, and she knew that she was in big trouble. She just sat there curled up in a ball with her eyes closed and waited.

As the stomping of her father's feet became louder, she cringed and started to shake. Then she heard her dad and mom viciously fighting in the other room. As their voices elevated, tears streamed down her face. She didn't know what to do. Lisa was so frightened that she wet her pants sitting in the darkness, as she shook and rocked. Her father's voice was so brutal and loud, and her mother's nasty tongue was sharp as a knife as she knew how to push every one of his buttons.

When the yelling was over, Lisa emerged from the closet. As she stood there with her pants all wet, the door to her room flew opened. He father entered, and she was terrified. He stood there, larger than life and angry as hell.

He then unleashed his anger and fear onto her. He never laid a hand on her but screamed at her until she wet her pants for a second time. The more Lisa cried, the more he yelled.

"What the fuck is wrong with you? You let this man in our house, and did you see he came back with a van? That was not for the furniture—that was for you! Do you hear me, *THAT WAS FOR YOU!* He came here to kidnap you, I know it! Oh my god, how stupid are you?" John was so beside himself, he began to shake, as his eyes bulged out of his head. He looked her in the eyes and yelled, "Don't ever, ever do that again! Do you hear me!"

Lisa put her head down and whispered,"Ok."

John walked out, slammed the door, and then Lisa heard him grab his keys and march out the front door. He took off like a bat out of hell down the street. Lisa just stood there and cried her eyes out. When she finally emerged from her room to get cleaned up, her mother came down the hall.

"Nice move asshole," was all that she said and went back into her room. She then proceeded to blare the music so loud that Lisa covered her ears!

Lisa went into the bathroom, cleaned herself up, and proceeded to lay on the couch to watch television. As she was laying there, barely able to hear the sound of the television over her mother's music, she started to recap her day in of her mind.

Dinner was never cooked that night so Lisa ate cereal alone as she thought about the creepy man.

*Was that man really going to steal me?* she thought to herself.

## Pretty Baby: When Things Would Turn Inappropriate

Joann had many friends. She hated to be home for too long, so she would always make plans to visit people. She had a childhood friend, Pat. Joann and Pat had a long history together, as they were best friends throughout their teen years, right on into adulthood.

They always stayed in touch, as they both married, and had children around the same time frame. There were many family gatherings together. After the passing of Jon, it was hard for Joann to visit Pat at times, because she had two beautiful healthy sons.

When Joann was in her manic state (the high), she would talk very quickly, and her thoughts would gravitate towards vulgar language and sexual innuendos. This is something she and Pat had in common when Joann was in this mode.

Pat also had her own highs and lows, and they would feed off of each other's energy and behaviors.

During one visit to Pat's home, there was an inappropriate incident that left Lisa quite upset.

It was a cold day in mid-January. There was snow on the ground, and the children did not have school. Lisa was happily playing alone in her room. At this time, she was twelve years old. Lisa loved to play with her Barbie dolls and spent countless hours with them, as her imagination took her to faraway places.

Her home had turned into a festering pool of dysfunction, and this was a great way to distract herself from the reality of her home life.

"Lisa, Lisa, come into the kitchen now!" yelled her mother.

Lisa rolled her eyes and pretended not to hear her, but she continued to bellow, so Lisa knew she had to go see what was going on.

As she stepped into the kitchen, there was her mother, sitting at the kitchen table. What a sight she was. Her hair was teased up extremely high, and her face was loaded with makeup. Her blue eye shadow was so bright and thickly applied, you could see it from down the hallway.

Lisa knew exactly what that meant. Her mother was off on a manic high again. Slowly she approached her mother, waiting to see what type of reaction she would get.

"Oh, look at you all in your room playing with your dolls. Were they fucking?"

Lisa's eyes grew wide and her tummy felt sick.

"C'mon Lisa, can't you take a joke?" Joann then laughed uncontrollably.

Lisa just stood there watching her mother become so big and animated, as the smoke from her cigarette floated out of her mouth.

"We are going to Pat's house. Go get yourself ready!"

"I do not want to go mom, I want to stay home and play."

"Well, we are not staying home. You can go play with the boys, maybe even kiss each other!" Joann said sheepishly with a big grin.

"Ew Mom stop! I don't kiss boys!" argued Lisa.

"You will someday and even have lots of sex! Should we talk about sex, Lisa?"

"*NO* mom, let's not; I will go get ready."

As Lisa turned to walk back down the hall, she could hear her mom singing crazy songs, and she just shook her head.

As they made their way outside, the snow was fairly deep, and the winter winds were blowing. The road was, slippery and the ride over to Pat's house was quite eventful. When Joann was revved up, she felt like she was on top of the world, and no snow storm was going to slow her down. She sped through the streets like a banshee, almost side-swiping a car or two along the way.

Lisa held on for dear life, terrified that they were going to get killed.

"Slow down mommy. You are driving too fast!"

"Don't tell me what to do you little bitch, I am in charge of this show!" protested Joann, who was now instantly angry.

She then proceeded to backhand Lisa across the face so hard, Lisa's head felt like it was spinning. She began to cry as Joann berated her for being such a baby.

This horrible scenario had become routine in Lisa's life, as Joann continued to spiral out of control over the past few years since her son's death. She would fall into deep depressions, be put on medications, and then she would take herself back off so she could feel the highs of life as she called them. Those highs (manic episodes) were dangerous on many levels.

They made it to Pat's house in one piece and were greeted at the door, with big smiles and warm hellos. Pat noticed the mark on Lisa's face and looked at her sympathetically, but did not acknowledge it.

Once inside, the energy level begans to heighten. The children were instructed to go to the playroom, and Pat brought them snacks and drinks.

Pat had two boys, Greg and Donny. Greg was the same age as Lisa, and Donny was two-years younger. As the kids happily played games together, Joann and Pat sat at the table drinking coffee and smoking cigarettes.

Lisa could hear her mother's uncontrollable laughter from the other room, but tried to ignore it. Her voice triggered so many emotions inside of Lisa, many of them she could not even describe or truly understand.

Greg turned to Lisa and said, "Boy your mom is crazy. I thought my mom was crazy, but your mom is much worse."

Lisa was annoyed and told him to shut up. Donny giggled at the two of them.

"Oh, isn't that sweet. The two love birds are fighting." Lisa turned her head in embarrassment, as it was her mother standing in the doorway. "Lisa, I have the best idea. Remember the movie, *Pretty Baby*, with Brooke Shields?"

"Yes, why?" asked Lisa.

"I have a great idea. Let's reenact the scene when they were getting her all washed up before she was sold and lost her virginity! Pat is running a bath for you right now with some bubbles. You said you always loved her bathtub. Now you get a chance to use it!"

Lisa was sickened by the thought of what was about to happen.

"NO, Mom, I am not doing that!" Lisa argued with her mother, adamant about not budging.

Joann marched over to her and demanded that she get up and go to the bathroom where she would strip down and get into the tub. The boys were looking at her mother in disbelief.

Lisa started to cry, "Mom, *please* don't make me do it!"

"You will do as I say right now! Let's go!"

Lisa got up slowly and made her way to the bathroom. She felt so sick, like she was going to throw up. She could hear her mother say to the boys, "You wait here. We will call you in when we are ready for you."

When Lisa stepped into the bathroom, her friend Pat had lit some candles and the essence of sexuality stunk up the place. These two women before her eyes were so emerged in the moment it was horrifying. Lisa was totally disgusted. They both chatted about the movie and instructed Lisa to get naked immediately to play out the scene. She silently did as she was told, as they continued to talk about her tight little body.

Lisa was humiliated and embarrassed as she quickly jumped in the tub filled with bubbles to hide herself. They both instructed her to wash herself, and Pat sprayed perfume in the air. It was a cross between rose petals and gardenias. It smelled beautiful, and she closed her eyes for a moment and began to float away. Their voices became distant to her, and it felt like she was walking amongst flowers in a beautiful field, as the sun shone brightly upon her. In this moment she felt total peace.

"Come on in boys for your viewing pleasure!" sang Joann in a loud voice, snapping Lisa back into the reality of her true situation.

When Lisa opened her eyes, not only were her mom and Pat standing in the bathroom, but now Greg and Donny were too. Lisa wanted to die right there, as the boys ogled her naked body with their eyes.

"Wow!" said Donny. "This is awesome!"

Greg, on the other hand, had the same embarrassed look on his face like Lisa did.

"Mom, I need to get out of here!" Greg stated.

"Now, now Greg. This is your future wife, and you will get to take her virginity! Look at your prize!" Joann stated proudly! "Do you want a quick feel of your future?"

"Mom stop, stop it!" Lisa screamed.

Greg ran out of the room, dragging his reluctant brother behind him.

"Ok, ok." said Pat. "I think we are done here for now. Let's let Lisa enjoy her bath."

Joann shot Lisa a look of displeasure but agreed with Pat. They went off into the other room, but before Pat shut the door, she peeked her head back in and said, "Lisa take as long as you would like sweetie." Then she closed the door.

Lisa was frozen in fear and furious at the same time. She did not want to move, but her anger burned as she could hear her mother's voice coming from the other room talking about big dicks and sex with Pat.

"Sure, enjoy my bath." Lisa said out loud, mocking these women who are supposed to protect her, not shame her and throw her to the wolves!

This incident left her traumatized, shamed and feeling extremely dirty.

*Note: The movie Pretty Baby was about a young girl who grew up in a house of prostitution and was auctioned off to the highest bidder. The first man to take her virginity. In the movie she was a 12-year-old girl.*

*That is exactly how Lisa felt in that moment.*

**The Sex Talk with Joann—**

When Joann was on an extreme high, her sexual personality would kick in. Lisa would be subjected to all sorts of sexual stories that were completely inappropriate and disgusting.

Lisa heard many stories of her own parents' sexual encounters, stories about the neighbors down the street, and everything else that her mom would come up with.

Not only did she hear about sex in general, she also heard about straight sex, gay sex, and domination. There was not a topic that was not up for grabs!

When Lisa would be in her playroom escaping into her own little fantasy world, her safe space so to speak, she would play with her baby dolls and Barbies. She loved taking them on so many adventures, and of course, all of them had happy endings.

Lisa tried desperately to shelter herself against the "Wrath of Joann" and learned when to stay away and hide. Most of these safe moments were short lived, because even though she would close the door, her mother would burst in with many words of distorted wisdom. Joann seemed to love to share these twisted ideals with Lisa, and she would become louder, animated, and aggressive when she spoke in such a way.

One day Joann came in as Lisa was sitting on the floor dressing her dolls. As her mom entered the room, she rolled her eyes and turned her head hoping it wouldn't be too brutal, but she was wrong.

Joann sat on the chair and asked her, "Are your dolls fucking each other today? Did Barbie show Ken her twat?"

Lisa shot her a disturbed look and bluntly stated, "*NO!* Stop Mom!"

Joann began to laugh hysterically and went on to taunt her daughter.

"Lisa, let me tell you a story because you need to know these things. You know Lorraine, Jenny's mom, right?"

"Yes mom of course I do, why?"

"I was talking to her the other day, and she was telling me how she gets ass fucked by her husband, and that is his favorite thing to do!"

Lisa's mouth dropped open as she could not believe the words that just came out of her mother's mouth. This was a new low.

"I told Lorraine that she is going to burn in hell if she continues to let him fuck her up the ass, because Jesus said "No Ass Fucking!" Do you hear me Lisa?" Joann rambled on as her voice became more intense.

"Yes, mom I hear you. Now please stop.".

Joann became agitated and forced Lisa to repeat what she said. "Say it Lisa, say it."Repeat what I just told you, so I know you heard me."

*"NO Mom!"*

"Say it you little bitch, or I will slap your face! NOW!" Joann screamed, hovering over her.

Lisa was a so sickened by her mother's behaviors but knew if she did not do what she was told, it would get so much worse, so she took a deep breath and stated, "No ass fucking. Jesus said." Lisa then swallowed her own saliva that was building up inside her mouth as she fought back tears. Her deep blue eyes were piercing at her mother in such contempt as her lip puckered a bit.

Joann stared her down with a psychotic look on her face and then burst out into uncontrollable laughter. She stood up and started to dance and sing wildly all-around Lisa, clapping her hands and kicking her feet. She poked Lisa a few times with her big toe and was taunting her for saying such dirty words.

Lisa curled up in a ball just waiting for it to be over.

When Joann had enough, she turned around and left the room just as quickly as she came in.

As Lisa sat there trying to process what had just happened, she shook uncontrollably. Then she got up, picked up her dolls, and put them all away. Joann ruined her innocence, and now Lisa felt the dolls were as dirty as her mother's behaviors. It was time to start packing them away.

After this incident and another incident in her home, Lisa was done. Joann invited a bunch of kids from Lisa's class to have a party. This was the night Joann encouraged the kids to play spin the bottle, and forced Lisa to kiss a boy!

Lisa did not want to kiss anyone but knew if she didn't, her mother would further embarrass her.

Her classmates then went on to make fun of her profusely for still having dolls. It was now game over. The last strands of her childhood innocence were gone forever.

The dolls were packed away the next day. Never to be played with again.

Lisa was a very sad and confused young girl, with internal anger that was beginning to build.

**Halloween Madness**

The holidays brought out many things in Joann, and for some reason, Halloween always seemed to put her over the top. Lisa was not sure about the connection as to why she behaved the way she did, or what the actual trigger was, but it was huge. Maybe she was feeding off of the energy that this holiday exuberated.

Joann would always dress up like Aunt Jemima and paint her face black with cork.

She would always use cork and only cork! She would tie a scarf around her head and put on a big moomoo dress. When her look was complete, she was ready for action. For some reason, she took great pleasure in dressing up as this character.

This insane ritual went on for many years as she behaved in such a horrid manner. She would think nothing of dropping the "N" word and drawing negative attention to herself. When other people would get angry or disgusted with her, she would become aggressive and wild. She would also scream, rant, and rave, literally scaring people away. Unfortunately, her daughter was always with her during these uncomfortable and embarrassing times.

Joann even showed up at her daughter's school dressed in such a way, sashaying down the hallway making crude remarks as she caused a big scene.

Finally, the principal asked her to leave, and of course, the other kids laughed, making fun of Lisa for having such a crazy mother. It was endless and extremely exhausting trying to keep up with her pace. There was always an incident that Lisa would have to try to explain to others, and sometimes there were just no words.

It was the year 1978, and Joann was at an all-time low. She was not taking any of her medications, and she was completely out of control. As Halloween approached, she had a different idea of what would play out for this season.

She decided that she and Lisa would both dress up as hookers and go driving around town before the Halloween party at the local roller-skating rink. Of course, Lisa did not want to dress up in such a way. Nor did she want to go anywhere with her crazy-ass mother, but she knew that she had no choice.

As her mother dressed her daughter in a provocative way, forcing her not to wear a bra and finishing off the look with dark red lipstick, Lisa was beside herself. Joann then put on her classic tube top and long skirt. She teased her hair up high and tied a bright orange scarf in her hair.

Joann was revved up and told Lisa that she needed to drive, because she wanted to really enjoy herself. At this time, Lisa was almost thirteen years old, and a professional driver, due to the fact that she was forced to learn at a young age. Her mother would have her drive all the time because she just didn't want to.

As they got into the big Pontiac Catalina, Joann was hooting and hollering at the neighbors. She was waving at them like she was a celebrity. Lisa quickly got into the car, and they drove off. The neighbor's all saw that Lisa was driving on a regular basis, but nobody ever said a word. This was a silent pattern of the neighborhood. It was like an "unspoken" pact that was made.

Joann instructed Lisa to drive down by the beach. As they pulled up to the light, there was a group of young men in the car next to them. Joann quickly rolled down the window and was yelling, "You want to see my tits?" and proceeded to pull down her tube top. The guys in the car were screaming many obscene things at her, and she seemed to relish every moment of it. As she waved her naked breasts out the window, it was like freedom for her. This caged animal was finally set free to roam aimlessly, doing anything she deemed necessary to fulfill her insatiable need for sexual attention.

Lisa was now screaming at her mother to stop and put the gas pedal to the floor, taking off like the speed of sound. Joann lurched back as the car took off. This car had power, and on that night, Lisa took advantage of it. There was no fear in her eyes, just contempt.

When they hit the next light, Joann blew up on her daughter, smashing her with her open hand about ten times. Lisa blocked her over and over again, taking each blow as it came. Finally, Joann stopped. She looked over and saw an old couple in the car next to them staring in horror. Joann flipped them the bird and yelled out the window, "What's the matter, you can't take a joke you old fuckers!"

Again, Lisa drove off down the road trying to get away from other vehicles, silently swearing in her head, using some of the many words that her mother had taught her over the years. Joann was laughing as she lit up a cigarette.

She looked over at her daughter and said, "Poor Lisa she just can't handle the fun."

Lisa remained quiet, ignoring her mother as they pulled into the roller-skating rink. Once they were parked, she let out a big sigh.

Joann got out and said, "Let's go and have some more fun."

"I will be there in a minute ok, mom?"

"Fine, but don't take too long. I will be looking for you," Joann said as she walked away.

Lisa just sat there with her two hands on the wheels thinking, "Yes, I know you will!"

As she watched her mom walk inside the building, she started to cry as she shook her head over and over again.

*Why ME?*

## The Cheerleader

Lisa had many secret ambitions for herself, and none of them included what life was handing her at this time. Lisa fought off the negativity like a soldier marching into battle every single day.

She had dreams, wishes, and many grand ideas for her future. She would write them all down in her journal and dream about a better life. One of her dreams was to become a cheerleader. Lisa always wanted to cheer and be a part of a team.

When her school announced that they were having cheerleading tryouts, Lisa was ecstatic! She thought this could be her chance to break free, be involved in something new and exciting. As Lisa gathered all the information about tryouts, she did not tell a soul, especially her mother.

When the day finally arrived, Lisa gave it all that she had and hoped for the best. The coaches loved her, and she was told that very day that she made the squad. She was over the moon with happiness. She jumped up and down with the other girls as they all chattered together. Even though it was junior high, Lisa felt so grown up as she said, "I am a cheerleader!"

When she arrived home that day, her mother was waiting for her at the kitchen table. At this time, they were now living with her grandparents because her parents were getting a divorce. Joann could not handle living on her own anymore, due to an incident when she did not arrive home one day after work. Lisa contacted her family members who came and got her as they searched for her mom. Unfortunately, her mom tried to commit suicide and was hospitalized. Lisa moved in with her father for a very short period of time but was returned back to her mother when she came home from the hospital.

"Where were you?" Joann snarled at her daughter.

"Well, mom I actually went out for the cheerleading squad and made it," Lisa said quietly.

"You did what? Who told you that you could do this?" Joann stated sounding quite annoyed.

"I told me to do it," Lisa said with a stark attitude. "It is something that I wanted to do, and I am doing it, I do not care what you think!" Lisa stood her ground.

Joann eyed her for a bit and said snidely, "OK big shot, that is fine, but I will be coming to all of your games!"

Lisa looked at her totally angry and raised her voice to her mother for the first time, "*NO* you are not! I don't want you there!"

"Well, if I am not there, then you will not be there either," Joann told her.

Lisa's heart sank into her stomach, as she silently turned and walked down the hallway to her room.

Joann remained in the kitchen taunting her as she walked away. "Boo Hoo, Mona Lisa is not happy! Too bad!"

The next day, Lisa started practicing. She decided to just go with it, telling herself it would be alright. She worked really hard, and when she received her uniform, she was so proud. She called her dad and asked him to please help her get her cheer sneakers because they had to be a certain brand. He was not too happy about it at first but then agreed to help her.

Lisa stood in the mirror as she put on her blue and white uniform. Her eyes shone brightly as she eyed herself, feeling so good from head to toe. It was all so perfect. She said to herself, *"You can do this!"* As she put the finishing touches on her look with a big blue bow in her hair, she felt so proud.

The next day was her first big game. Her mother forced her to give her the schedule, and Lisa cringed hoping that she would not come. When school ended that day, all the girls went to the gym and changed into their uniforms. It was such a happy moment. Lisa felt like she actually belonged. As they all got onto the bus . . . football players, cheerleaders, and coaches . . . , the energy was high, filled with such excitement.

The first game was a great success. Lisa cheered her heart out, was part of a cheerleading pyramid, and the boys won! The best part of the day was that her mom was a no-show, but unfortunately, so was her dad. Lisa invited him, but he did not come.

As she rode the bus home from the game, many thoughts went through her mind. There was a bit of sadness that filtered through the excitement. As they pulled into the school and proceeded to get off of the bus, many kids were greeted by their parents with smiles, hugs, and kisses. As everyone went to their vehicles, Lisa gathered up her belongings, changed into her other sneakers, and started her long walk home with her pom poms in hand.

There was nobody there for her, and she accepted that because she was finally able to do something that she enjoyed. She kept telling herself nobody was going to stop her. When she got home, her grandparents were there in the kitchen and asked her how it went. Lisa shared her joy about cheering and winning the game. Her grandparents seemed genuinely happy for her. She then asked her grandmother where her mom was.

"Lisa, she has not left her room all day," Rose sighed.

"Ok, then," Lisa responded.

She knew she had to go in there to get her clothing, as they shared a room. Lisa also knew that the room would be filled with smoke, which she detested more than anything.

Lisa went in quickly, grabbed her things, and walked back out. Her mother was extremely quiet. She didn't even acknowledge her daughter's presence. Lisa was sad and thankful at the same time.

Lisa managed to get through her first few games without her mom in attendance and felt maybe it would be ok after all, until one day it just wasn't.

As the bus pulled up to the game, Lisa spotted her mother leaning against her car. She froze for a moment, and her friends asked her what was wrong.

"Nothing, nothing, there is my mom," Lisa said.

The girls looked over and just made a face toward Lisa. Of course, Joann was standing there with outlandish clothing (dressed like a gypsy), bright pink lipstick, and she was smoking.

When she saw Lisa, she started yelling, "Lisa, Lisa, there is my baby! Look at her, isn't she beautiful!"

Everyone was looking, and she was totally embarrassed. Lisa ran over to her mom to try to talk to her, but the coach called her back over. Lisa took her place, and the game began.

Every time they began to cheer, Joann cheered with them. She decided to come up closer and stood behind the line, yelling and screaming. Then she felt the need to take it up a notch and added vulgarity to the cheers.

"Let's go Big Blue. Let's fuck them up! Shake your asses, show your tits girls! Show these boys what you got!"

The coach was appalled and went over to speak to her.

Joann immediately got aggressive calling her all sorts of names including a "cunt." She made a huge scene. Lisa was so mortified, and some of the kids were pointing and laughing as Joann made a total spectacle of herself.

The coach walked over to Lisa and said, "You need to leave with your mother immediately. We cannot have this on our squad, so I am sorry you have to go."

Lisa was heartbroken and shocked that the coach would cut her and was more disturbed that she was sending her off with her mother at that very moment.

*Why do I have to be responsible for my mother's awful behaviors?*

*Why am I supposed to be the one to take care of her, she is supposed to take care of me?*

*Why am I always punished because of her?*

*I hate her!*

These were all the thoughts going through Lisa's head.

Lisa remained silent as she put her head down and walked away, but inside she was screaming *DOESN'T ANYONE SEE, DOESN'T ANYONE CARE? HELP ME!*

As she walked to the car, one of her friends grabbed her hand and said, "I'm sorry." Then ran back to the squad.

Lisa got in the car, and her mother was still cursing and screaming as they drove off. She was beeping the horn and giving them all the finger. Lisa sunk down in the seat, and her mother screamed at her the whole way home.

That was the beginning and end of Lisa's cheerleading dream. The next day she went to see the coach and handed her back the uniform. The coach just said she was sorry and that was it. Lisa was never asked if she was ok, or safe in her home; absolutely nothing was acknowledged. As Lisa left the gymnasium, some of the other girls were being very mean, pointing and whispering. Lisa heard them as they chuckled. It was quite hurtful. There were a couple of girls that talked to her briefly before she left, but they never continued on with the friendship because she was off the squad.

Back to square one.

## Aliens and Burning Bushes

Joann fought her demons and anyone else who got in her way! This meant that Joann fought the system. A system that had failed her on so many levels. The one thing that her doctors and therapists did agree upon was that Joann needed her medications to function appropriately.

After she tried to commit suicide and did a stint in the psychiatric unit, she was released to her parents. Joann and Lisa moved in, and this small house up on the hill was filled to the brim with many different types of personalities and dysfunctions—with nowhere to hide.

Lisa was forced to share a room with her mother. This was quite difficult for her as no teen should have to share a space with their parent, especially a sick parent. Joann took over the room with her loud music, constant smoking, and bed wetting from her continual cough. These two co-existed on the most dysfunctional and volatile level. Joann was severely mentally ill, and Lisa was a damaged, angry teen. Many altercations happened in that room over time.

Now, let's add in the fact that Joann once again decided to take herself off of her mediation, because she felt she did not need them anymore.

"Mom why are you not taking your pills? They help you," Lisa stated.

"I am allergic to those stupid pills. They make me sick. I want to feel, and they make my head buzz," Joann answered.

"Then tell the doctor and see what else they could give you to try, but you cannot stay like this," Lisa bantered.

"Don't you tell me what to do, you little bitch. I will smash your face." Joann was now cross.

"I hate you, you crazy bitch, I wish you were dead!" Lisa screamed back at her.

Joann got up from her chair, but her mother chimed in, "Joann, sit back down and leave her alone. Do you hear me?" Rose was angry. "Lisa, stop talking to your mother like that, now go find something to do!" Lisa looked at her grandmother and just let out a ferocious scream in frustration, then proceeded to storm out of the house.

As she was walking away, she heard her mother yelling out the door at her! "Lisa, Lisa, watch out for those aliens! Do you see them right in front of you?"

Lisa turned around annoyed and disgusted at the same time. Taking a deep breath, Lisa yelled, "There are no fucking aliens out here mom! Go inside!" Lisa then turned back around and kept on walking as her mother continued to bellow at her until she was out of sight.

From that day forward, things progressively got worse. The downward spiral had begun. No medication for Joann meant— voices, hallucinations, aggressive behaviors, violence, and many tears. There was no talking to her when she was in this state of mind. You cannot reason with "crazy," right?

When Joann hit rock bottom from this latest boycott of her medications, it was truly a horrid scene. She was now seeing aliens flying across the sky, several of them. She would jump up and run to the window freaking out, banging on the glass, screaming obscenities at her visions. This was a repeat performance for days on end.

Then there was the burning bush . . .

Joann was devoutly religious, and when she was in her balanced state of mind, she expressed her love for God and faith. She really did have a very strong belief system and prayed every single day.

When Joann was off of her medications, it was a whole different type of picture for her. She cursed like a sailor, used such sexual vulgarity that the hair would singe off of your eyebrows, and she spoke of the devil. Joann would also curse at God and Jesus for forsaking her with such internal pain and blamed the devil for playing such cruel tricks on her.

As Joann wandered the house creating havoc in every room that she went into, she made her way back to the kitchen. Lisa was sitting there talking to her grandmother when Joann entered the room.

"Did you see him go by?" Joann asked.

"Who mom?" asked Lisa.

"The devil. He just ran past my bedroom door; he is taunting me again."

"No mom, he is not here, go back to what you were doing," Lisa said, annoyed.

Joann ran over to the door and immediately started screaming. "Look, look the bush is burning, and the flames are wrapping around Mother Mary and the baby Jesus! We need to help them!"

Rose was instantly up in arms; not quite sure what to do. Rose was blind, so you could only imagine how hard it was for her to visualize what Joann was doing. Lisa jumped into action and tried to stop her mom from going out of the door.

"Mom, Mom, its ok that is not real. Look at it again it is not real!" Lisa yelled in a panic.

Joann was screaming, Lisa was screaming, and now Rose was screaming because she didn't want Joann leaving the house in such a state.

"That devil, he is after me, he is after me! I am going to kill him!" Joann was shrieking at the top of her lungs! Then, Joann picked up Lisa and tossed her out of the way as she ran out the door.

"Lisa hurry, go get her!" Rose said in a panicked tone.

As Lisa ran out of the door, her uncle was coming up the driveway with his wife, and he intervened with the situation at hand. He did not know the nature of what was happening, but he knew all too well that the best thing that should happen was to get her back inside the house. He could see the panic on Lisa's face.

Joann was completely out of control, but he managed to get her back inside with a lot of coercing. Once they were back in the house, another explosion began. Joann's brother had a very hard time understanding or communicating with her, so he said foolish things at times, which agitated the situation even more. When his wife stepped in to offer advice, Joann lunged at her, grabbing her by the shoulders, picking her up, and proceeding to toss her across the room.

She was devastated and completely frightened, so she started crying. This is when her husband stepped in to save her from his sister's wrath. She now turned her anger toward him and began to hit him repeatedly. He blocked her over and over again, never striking back, but he tried to shield himself from Joann's hurricane of fury. Lisa stood there frozen, as she had been on the end of that fist countless times before.

Finally, Joann calmed down a bit, because she could hear her own mother crying. Joann loved her mother fiercely, so the thought of bringing her to that point triggered something inside of her. Joann stepped away from her brother and just stared blankly at him. She looked like a statue completely frozen. It was a huge mess, and there seemed to be no end—and no way out.

Lisa remained silent as the adults bantered back and forth, as Joann turned around, finally retreating to her room.

"Lisa, give me the phone and dial your aunt's number for me." Rose instructed in a distressed tone.

Rose knew during these difficult times that her daughter would step in and call the doctor for advice. As Lisa dialed the phone, she was shaking. Once the phone started ringing, she handed it to her grandmother, as she was still unable to speak.

"Hello, it's mom. Joann is out of control again, and she just attacked your brother and his wife. I need you to call the doctor immediately. She needs to go back to the hospital." Rose was quite clear in her instructions.

Her daughter replied with, "Ok mom. I am on it."

What transpired after that phone call was pure madness. The doctor instructed them to bring her into the clinic as soon as possible. Once Joann was there, they would call for the police and an ambulance for transport to the hospital.

It was a horrible scene at the clinic. Joann walked in and immediately created a scene. She was larger than life in that moment, but they managed to corral her, as she was instantly ushered into the backroom. Lisa and her aunt followed along silently.

The doctor came in and tried to have a conversation with her, which instantly went sour in about two seconds flat.

Joann immediately screamed at him, that they were not taking her to the fucking hospital, and there was nothing wrong with her. She became so explosive that she started to throw items at him. He stepped out of the room as they tried to calm her down.

A few minutes later the police walked in, and the EMTs were behind them. Joann instantly went into fight mode. She was ranting and screaming like a lunatic, "You will not take me alive! I will kill you all!" The police wasted no time in engaging in a brutal struggle as they wrestled her to the floor. Joann had the strength of ten men when she was manic. She would not give up without a fight!

Lisa and her aunt watched in horror and dismay as this display unfolded before their eyes. This left them feeling helpless and angry at the same time. They wanted to step in and help her, but there was nothing they could do but stand there and watch as the battle raged on.

Lisa started crying hysterically and that is when Joann calmed down.

Joann started yelling, "My daughter! My daughter! Look what you are doing to my baby girl! STOP—STOP—STOP!"

Lisa cried out, "Mom, please go with them, stop fighting now, let them help you!" Lisa was sobbing profusely as she dropped to the floor.

Joann agreed to stop fighting. The police brought her to her feet and helped her carefully onto the stretcher. As the EMTs were strapping her in, she spat at the police officers and called them all sorts of obscenities. Joann then turned her attention to her sister and daughter, who was now back on her feet.

"You two are to blame for all of this, I hope you are happy. You are cowards, do you hear me, cowards!"

Lisa's aunt was silent, but Lisa approached her mom and said, "I am sorry mom, but you need to get better."

"Fuck you bitch. You're dead to me now!" Joann growled with contempt.

Lisa put her head down and stepped back, and they proceeded to wheel her down the hallway as she screamed and threatened everyone all the way out the door.

Lisa's aunt spoke with the doctor about what the procedures were and then turned back to Lisa and said, "Let's go home."

The ride back up to the house was silent. They were both mentally exhausted from the experience. Once they were back home, Lisa retreated to her room.

She then did what worked for her during these stressful times, she cleaned! She spent hours in there scrubbing and cleaning every inch of that room. She scrubbed as she talked to herself, as she tried to wrap her head around everything that was going on.

When she was finally done, she just laid on the bed completely exhausted. She was intensely smelling the cleanliness of the sheets and blankets with pure delight. As she took it all in the day . . . the room, the smells . . ., she suddenly felt sleepy.

As she dosed off, she could hear the words of her mother:

**"YOU ARE DEAD TO ME, THIS IS ALL YOUR FAULT!"**

She fought off the sounds of her mother's voice, knowing she needed rest before her mom returned back home. As Lisa laid there feeling weak, she thought about how much alone time she would have in this room before her mom would come back to create more havoc on her and the family. She winced at the thought of it all but embraced the silence, as she fell fast asleep.

# Chapter 12

# The Battle Of The Wills— Mother vs Daughter

In the last chapter, the combined short stories were just a few of the many incidents and experiences that transpired over the years after the passing of Joann's son. This shows her downward spiral and continued struggles that faced her every single day. These short stories also display the effects that her illness played upon her husband, daughter, and family.

Over the course of that time, Joann also struggled with so many insecurities about illness and death, especially when it came to her own daughter. Every time Lisa became ill with a cold, virus, or bacterial infection as all kids do, it was a major experience.

Joann would go into an instant panic mode, as her thoughts would shift directly to the dark side, as she always thought her child was deathly ill. This is what would transpire in her clouded mind. She would call the pediatrician, hysterical all the time, and would rush her daughter in to be examined immediately. Dr. Morris was very kind to her, and all of the nurses for the most part were too, except for one whom seemed to dislike her very much. She always gave Joann an attitude, and Joann seemed to trigger the nurse for some unapparent reason.

Joann and Nurse Sue had many verbal confrontations over the years, and some of the words that were used, were not kind, that was for sure. Lisa was always a part of these negative encounters, and it disturbed and embarrassed her greatly.

Nurse Sue would always look at Lisa and say, "Are you ok?"

Lisa would always reply, "Yes."

That was the extent of any outside help for Lisa in regards to support from her doctor's office. Dr. M knew very well of Joann's issues, but he never asked Lisa anything in regards to her well-being or safety. This scenario has to make you think about what if Nurse Sue made some direct comments to the doctor about Lisa's safety, and was immediately shut down (Another sign of the times—never ask questions—never speak of such things).

With Joann being so paranoid about illness, blood tests, and vaccinations, Lisa was excluded from many things. There was never a flu vaccination, blood tests for any reason, and the tonsils that were plagued with strep infection over and over again remained, because Joann refused to let Lisa have the surgery. In her heart, she felt Lisa would die.

This is a part of the illness that overtook Joann completely, and in her mind, there was death and doom everyday. Joann fought everyone in her path to get her way, and she refused to back down, especially when it came to Lisa's health and what she thought was best for her. It was a very twisted and distorted view for her, and Lisa suffered the consequences of her actions and decisions.

As Lisa got older, she became a bit defiant. The years of repeated abuse had taken a toll on her, and she was ready to fight back. It came slowly, and in stages, but it was now coming to the surface—the internal rage, detest and contempt for all that she had been through at the hands of her own mother.

It was the fall of 1979, and school was back in session. Joann was at an extreme low because of her divorce from her husband, the transition back to her parents' home, and the daily battle inside her own mind.

As Lisa made her way out the door, Joann would rattle off a list of paranoid worries, thoughts, and fears. Lisa would brush them off the best she could because she tried not to have confrontations with her mother that early in the morning. Joann made it nearly impossible for her daughter to remain quiet, and many times the battle of words would ignite.

The fury of mother and daughter began to rage on almost daily!

When Lisa finally made it out the door, she breathed a sign of relief, because now she could really begin her day. Lisa walked to school every day. Sometimes it would be alone, or other times with a few friends. It was quite a far walk, but she didn't mind as long as she was away from home.

## Science Class—1979

Lisa made her way back home and slowly trudged up the big hill, contemplating what would happen when she got there. As she made her way through the door, her grandmother was the first to greet her. Lisa always knew that her grandmother would be sitting at the kitchen table drinking her coffee.

"How was your day?" she asked.

"It was a good day grandma and guess what?" Lisa responded. "I was in science class, and we are doing this really cool experiment. We are studying blood types, and we all get to have a test done to see what our blood type is!"

"Oh, that does sound fascinating Lisa," her grandmother replied. Rose was a highly intelligent woman and loved to learn and study about new things. She always enjoyed hearing about Lisa's studies because she was learning alongside her as well.

"I am excited about it."

Her words were cut off by her mother coming into the room. Lisa turned around to see her mom standing there.

"What blood test? Who is having a blood test? NOT you!" Joann snarled.

"Mom, it is an experiment in science class, and I am really excited about it. Can you please just sign the paper so I can be a part of it?" Lisa begged.

"Absolutely NOT!" Joann screamed on top of her lungs. "I will not have my daughter be poked with needles like your brother was! Don't you remember, you were there!"

"Yes, I remember all too well, but this is different and I am doing it!" Lisa retaliated back.

"You will not, and don't you dare tell me what you are going to do. I am the boss! Do you hear me!" Joann was instantly in a fury.

"I don't care what you say *MOM*, I am doing it! You, are not the boss of me!" Lisa was now staring her mother down as the rage was boiling inside of her.

*SLAP*—that was the sound Rose heard, then followed by a scream from Lisa, "I hate you, I hate you, you ruin everything in my life!" Then Rose heard footsteps pounding down the hall and into the laundry room where Lisa locked herself in.

"Joann!" Rose yelled, "What is the matter with you? Let that girl do what she needs to do. It is for school."

"I don't care what it is for. She will die if they stick her with a needle. They will give her leukemia, and she will die!" Now Joann was hysterically crying and cursing God for taking her only son, and the devil who was now trying to claim her daughter.

Joann went stomping down the hall, punched the door to the laundry room, and she screamed, "You will obey me or die!" Then she went back to her bedroom and slammed the door.

Lisa was sitting on the floor of the small laundry room, stuck. She was wedged between the dryer and the wall. As she was crying, she also began to shake profusely. As the tears ran down her face, she could feel the sting and burning from the hands of her mother. Then she heard a knock on the door.

"Lisa it is me, please come out," said Rose.

Lisa did not answer her. She sat for a long time, and when she finally emerged making her way back to the kitchen, her grandmother asked her if she was ok.

"Yes, I am fine," was all Lisa managed to mutter out.

Lisa tried to reapproach the subject over the next few days, but it was shot down. She left the paper on the table hoping her mother would sign it, but that did not happen. The morning of the science experiment, Lisa did not want to go to school, but she knew she had to. As she walked out the door, she was mad as a hornet, but remained completely silent. The last thing she heard as she closed the door was, "You better not defy me you little bitch!"

Lisa ignored her mom and slammed the door.

As she walked into science class, the kids were all excited about the experiment. It was middle school, eighth grade, and everyone was loud and boisterous. Lisa dropped in her seat looking cross. The teacher came over to her and asked where her permission slip was because she was the only one in the entire class without one.

Lisa explained that her mother refused to sign the form. The teacher proceeded to tell her that she could not participate in the experiment and would get a zero for the class project. This infuriated her even more, and she looked at her teacher and said, "That's Great!"

The teacher walked away and began to gather all of the other students together when there was a knock on the door, followed by a voice Lisa knew all too well. It was her mother! Lisa remembered that she left the paper on the table, and it had the date on it about the experiment. Her stomach flipped.

"May I help you?" The teacher asked, surprised to see her standing there.

"I am Lisa's mother, and how dare you want to stick her with a needle! You will give her leukemia, you, stupid prick!" Joann unleashed her vile rage onto him.

Mr. C was caught off guard and then proceeded to make his way toward her, yelling at her to leave the classroom immediately!

As they went out into the hall, he closed the door, but you could hear them yelling at each other. Some of the other students began to make fun of Lisa and laughed at her, calling her mother all sorts of names. Lisa sank in the chair and started to cry. Her friend sat next to her, tried to comfort her. There is not a whole lot of kindness and compassion in middle school, and Lisa was feeling it big time.

As the teacher made his way back into class, he said, "Lisa your mother was just escorted out, and you need to leave at once. I cannot have you in this classroom today. Go report to the principal. He is waiting for you."

"I do not want to go," Lisa said quite gruff and angry.

"You do not have a choice! Go now!" Mr. C replied.

"Yes, Lisa, go! We don't want you in here, because you are crazy like your mother!" Dee yelled out.

Lisa turned to here and screamed, "Shut the fuck up, you ugly douchebag!"

Mr. C said, "That is it, I have had enough. Lisa you have detention."

"Fuck you, Mr. C. Go shit in your hat," Lisa screamed and

marched out the door, slamming it shut.

*Fuck Everyone*, she thought to herself as she made her way to her locker. She grabbed her belongings and left the school. As she walked down the street, she was crying. Then a car pulled up alongside of her, and it was her mother.

"Get into this car at once! Do you hear me?" Joann yelled.

"NO mom! Go fuck yourself, you crazy bitch!" Lisa retaliated.

Joann started beeping the horn over and over again. "Get in this car NOW!"

People were starting to take notice, so Lisa got into the car, because she did not want any further attention brought to her.

"How dare you show up at my science class!" Lisa said, again challenging her mother.

"Don't you talk to me like that. I will punch you in the face!" Joann replied with one hand on the wheel and the other a clenched fist waving in Lisa's face.

"Go ahead, who gives a shit," Lisa replied.

Joann hit the pedal to the floor and drove like a mad woman all the way home, cursing and swearing the whole way. Lisa just sat there and took it all in. When they pulled in the driveway, she jumped out of the car and made her way into the house before her mom.

She was like a tornado coming through the door, and she began to yell at her grandmother.

"I hate that bitch! Do you hear me, I hate her! She came to my school and embarrassed the shit out of me, and now I am in trouble because of her!" Lisa was furious.

Joann made her way through the door, and the battle began. Lisa and Joann went at it.

"I wish you would die!" Lisa repeated those words over and over again with tears in her eyes.

Joann made her way towards her, chasing her around the kitchen table, trying to get a hold of her!

Rose was screaming at the two of them to stop it. Joann's father came down the hallway to intervene as he grabbed his daughter. "Lisa, go, get out of here now. Go!"

Lisa climbed under the table and ran down the hallway to the bathroom and proceeded to lock herself in.

She could hear her mother and grandfather battling. Lisa

jumped into the tub and covered her ears, as she rocked back and forth. She felt like she could not breathe as the sweat was pouring off of her face and forehead. She felt so hot and sick to her stomach. She then threw up in the toilet and just sat on the cool floor waiting for the madness to stop.

When all was finally quiet, Lisa came out of the bathroom. Her grandmother was waiting for her. Lisa sat at the table next to her.

"Lisa, you cannot fight with your mother like that. Do you hear me?" Rose stated.

Lisa looked at her in annoyance and mumbled, "OK".

That was the end of that conversation!

As the day came to a close, Lisa refused to sleep in her room because she had to share it with the person she hated most in life, so she chose to sleep on the couch.

The next day she got up, got herself together, and made her way off to school to find out her fate from the disaster of the day before.

Joann taunted her daughter during breakfast, but Lisa remained silent.

It became a theme for mother and daughter: Explosions and Silence.

# Chapter 13

# The Fury Raged On

For mother and daughter, the teen years proved to be quite challenging as the up and down battles raged on. The fighting was a daily occurrence with many battles resulting with physical altercations.

As Joann would pound her daughter's head against the wall, they would bounce all the way down the hallway like a pinball being knocked around out of control. Lisa would do anything to survive these battles including blocking, pushing, and fighting for her life. The one thing she did not do, was hit her mother back! Joann's inner beast could not be contained at times, and it was a scary place to be—the ladder of mental illness at its worst.

**Moments of Clarity**

Joann would have moments of clarity, and during these times her deepest, darkest depression would hit.

She would lay on her bed smoking and crying profusely. She would listen to the radio and connect with songs like "Sad Eyes," which would further fuel her depression. As she would lay there, she would think about how much she loved her family, especially her daughter, and she could not believe how mean and brutal she was to all of them.

During these moments, she would feel so helpless and low, falling into deep despair. The depression was her reality as it was speaking to her wanting to be acknowledged.

*"NO mania = Reality and Depression"*

This was very difficult for her to face. A very hard pill to swallow! The truth about herself and her illness were too much to bear. These thoughts made her so sad, realizing her lack of control and inner rage. As she pondered her thoughts, she would smoke her days away, lost in the shadows of her mind. She was numb to the world and could not get beyond herself during these distraught hours.

Joann would lay in bed for days, barely getting up. She had no urge to live or engage in life. She would refuse to eat or shower, and she would sit in her own pee. The bedroom that Lisa was forced to share with her mother would reek of urine and stale cigarettes.

Lisa could not even stand the thought of her mother being in such a state of mind and body. It made her internally crazy.

Lisa would shift emotional gears during these periods in her life. She would go from hatred of her mother to pity and sadness. The overall effect of Joann's illness had on her was over-whelming, and it clouded her thoughts.

Lisa would try to find ways to get her mother to engage in life again. Asking her mom to get up and please help herself, which was mostly rejected with venomous words that cut like a knife. Lisa refused to give up and went back for more, over and over again trying to get a different response.

This sick dysfunctional game would go on for weeks, and then just like a cool breeze, the tides would change. Joann would emerge from her darkness and come out swinging.

Once again, she had taken herself off of her medications and stopped seeing the doctors. The downward spiral would happen so quickly. In the blink of an eye, Joann would flip a switch.

She was now up and moving. She had gone from a slow-paced mumble, to a fast-paced manic chatter. Joann would speak so quickly at times you could barely understand a word that she was saying.

**Then it came, the personality switch.**

Joann was up early, showered, and dressed for the day. Lisa and her grandmother sat at the table having coffee and breakfast before Lisa headed off to school. She looked up to see her mother sashaying down the hallway into the kitchen.

"Good morning bitches, what is going on in here, any good dick talk?"

"Mom shut up," Lisa said disgusted.

"Haha, poor Mona Lisa, she cannot take a joke," Joann taunted her.

Before Rose could speak up, Lisa angrily answered her mother! "Mom I hate when you talk like that and look how you are dressed. You look like a nasty whore!"

"Lisa!" Rose interjected.

"Sorry grandma, but you should see her in her tube top and skirt, with that nasty red lipstick and blue eyeshadow!"

"Lisa, you're just jealous because you don't look this good and cannot land a man like I can. That is my goal today, to get some action!" Joann was in a mood.

"Joann, stop it at once!" Rose piped up, totally disgusted by the whole conversation.

"Yeah, yeah mom. Take everyone's side but mine as always," Joann rambled on in her fast-paced tone as she continued to taunt both her mother and daughter.

"I am off to school. I am out of here," Lisa announced as she got up, grabbed her things, and ran out the door. She could hear her mother's laughter as she made her way down the driveway.

When Joann was in this mindset, she was a force to be reckoned with. There was no stopping or controlling her behaviors. Her language was dirty, sexual, and disgusting. She would behave in such a provocative manner. The worst part of all of it was she did not see herself that way.

During her manic times, she was on top of the world. She would ride that psychotic energy wave until she would flatline. There was always a crash, and everyone just held their breath waiting for it to happen.

This particular emotional crash came very quickly, as Joann

made her way to the fire station next to our home and became sexually aggressive with a few of the firemen that were hanging around out front.

"Hey guys, aren't you all looking fine today. Who want to go a few rounds with me?" Joann was speaking in her sexiest voice. She went on to flirt, even pulling her tube top down for the boys to take a look! It was a horrific scene, and the firefighters were trying to get Joann to return home. They all knew her over there because in her moments of promiscuous behaviors, they were easy prey, as they were just a stone's throw away.

When they rejected her advances, she became verbally abusive and then violent. She flicked her lit cigarette at one of the fire fighter's spewing such vulgarity.

When they had enough of her vulgar and outlandish behaviors, they called the police.

Joann was taken away in handcuffs, kicking and screaming, fighting the whole way.

They brought her directly to the hospital for a psychological evaluation.

One of the firefighters walked over to deliver the disastrous news to Joann's parents, and when Lisa got home from school, they shared with her what happened.

Lisa was again embarrassed of her mother's behaviors and disgusted by what she did. She also felt sadness because her mom could never be just a mom. So many thoughts and feelings were running through her mind, and she knew she would have to go see her.

Joann was transferred to the psychiatric unit at Yale New Haven Hospital. Lisa called her father to share what happened and asked him if her could give her a ride down to New Haven. Her father reluctantly agreed.

The ride to New Haven was mostly silent and awkward. John was deep in thought and so was Lisa. Here it is, father and daughter so close, yet so far, not knowing how to communicate at all. There was so much that they both wanted to say, but the words would not come out. Lisa watched out the car window as they traveled along, just hoping that her mother was ok.

Lisa and her father made their way into the building, but when it came to going into the unit, that was solely on her.

"Lisa I cannot go in there. I will wait for you here." John said to his daughter.

"Dad, seriously, you are sending me in there alone?" Lisa was disappointed.

"Lisa if I go in there, it will make things worse. She will get even more crazy," he sighed.

Lisa thought to herself, and he was right. She would flip out at the sight of him.

"Ok dad I get it, wish me luck."

"If she gets to be too much, just walk out," John instructed her.

"Ok dad I will," Lisa responded with a sad tone.

Lisa hit the buzzer.

"Hello," a voice came through the speaker.

"Hello it is Lisa; I am here to see my mother, Joann."

The loud buzzing noise went off, and in she went, holding her breath. As the loud clank of the door hit behind her, she felt sick to her stomach.

As Lisa slowly made her way to the nurse's station, the image of all the patients sitting around in a circle, smoking, and talking was etched in her mind from previous visits. As she was making her way closer, those past images now became a reality! There were also many patients strapped into their chairs screaming for help. This song of sadness was consuming, and she felt it all the way through to the core of her soul. Lisa was scared, very scared, but she put on her game face when she spoke to the nurse.

"Hello, I am Lisa, and I am here to visit my mother, Joann."

"Are you here alone? How old are you?" the nurse asked.

"My dad is waiting for me outside the door. He did not want to upset my mother any further than she already is. They are divorced." Lisa said flatly. "I am 15 years old, and this is not my first rodeo," Lisa went on to say with a bit of an attitude. The nurse eyed her for a bit and said to follow her.

"Your mother is in here," the nurse said and pointed to her room. Lisa entered the room, already knowing what she would face.

"Mom, it's Lisa. I am here."

Lisa stood quietly waiting for a response. Joann turned around. She had a black eye and her makeup was smeared all over her face. Her once bright red lipstick was now stretched across her face, and she looked like a sadistic clown, as her eyes were bulging out of her head.

"Lisa, look what they did to your mother! They beat me and raped me, all those motherfuckers!" Joann was now spitting on the floor.

"Mom nobody raped you," Lisa said to her.

"Yes, they did. All of those firefighters gang banged me, and I was screaming for help and nobody came!" Joann starts to cry.

"Mom listen, that is not what happened. You got arrested for harassing them." Lisa tried to explain the reality, but Joann would not hear it.

She started screaming louder and louder about rape, torture, anal sex, and beatings. Lisa stood in horror not knowing what to say or do, and then Joann went on to point to a window that was not there, telling her about the children being molesting in there. She was begging Lisa to help them. (This theme of the children in the window was one that stayed consistent for Joann every time she went to the hospital).

"Mom, it is ok. The children are safe," Lisa said strongly.

"No, no, they are not! Look again, you have to believe me!" Joann screamed at her daughter.

The nurse came in to try to calm her down, and Joann went ballistic. As the nurse ran back out of the room to get help, Lisa tried to connect with her mother.

"Mom you have to listen to me. Please calm down, please for me!" Lisa was begging her. "I will save the children. I promise you! I promise it will be fine."

"Go now, do you hear me, go now save them Lisa! You are their only hope, DO YOU HEAR ME!" Joann screamed so violently, she peed all over the floor. Then the orderlies came bursting in the door, three of them with the nurse in tow. They forcefully pinned her down as the nurse injected her with Haldol. Lisa was leaning back against the wall as tears began to flow, sickened by this sight before her eyes, feeling helpless.

"STOP, YOU'RE HURTING HER!" Lisa directed her anger at the orderlies. "You have her under control. Now let her go! I mean it!" Lisa was furious!

The nurse turned around and said, "You have to leave now, let's go."

"I am not leaving until I say good-bye to my mother," Lisa was standing her ground.

"Make it quick," the nurse replied.

As the orderlies made their way by her, Lisa mumbled "assholes" and made her way over to her mother who was now laying across the bed even more disheveled.

"Mom, I am so sorry. I will save the children, ok? Please rest and get better. I love you," Lisa said. She was leaning in close to her mom as she talked because the drugs hit hard and quickly.

Joann was half awake, but she could hear her daughter's voice.

"Thank you Lisa. The children need you. I love you too," Joann mumbled as she fell asleep.

Lisa kissed her on the forehead, rubbed her arm, and just stood there for a moment saying a silent prayer over her lifeless mother. A small tear dripped from her eye as she heard the nurse summon her to leave the room.

Lisa walked out of the room once again devasted and defeated because she could not help her mother. The nurse said to her, "She will be alright. Let us take care of her now."

"Sure, take care of her, like those orderlies did, wrestling her down like that! She is a human being, you know," Lisa was snide.

The nurse was a bit taken aback by Lisa's comment and said, "How old are you again?"

"I am old enough to know better," Lisa replied and walked out the door.

She was thankful to see her dad standing there waiting for her, and she ran over to him and hugged him tight. He held his baby girl and said, "It will be alright."

As they walked down the hall, John asked her what happened in there. Lisa told him she did not want to talk about it. He took her hand, and they walked out of the hospital together. What he could not give her in words, she felt through the squeezing of her hand. She knew he loved her, but she needed more, so much more. The ride back home was silent. When they pulled in the driveway, Lisa kissed her dad goodbye and went into the house. As she listened to his car pull away, she did not turn around to watch him, because she did not want him to see her crying.

After all she was the tough one, right?

# Chapter 14

# Catch Me If You Can

As time moved forward, there were many moments of chaos as Joann fought her demons. There were countless hospital trips, long battles, and disappearing acts!

Joann was determined to live life her way, and on her terms, even if that meant defying everything that was seemingly logical and just. Joann had many different personalities, and she played each part to a tee. The theatrics were award winning to say the least, and if there was an award to be given, she would have won! The "I am crazy as fuck" Award seemed fitting in the moment!

During this time frame in her life, Joann and Lisa were still living in Joann's parents' home. They all rode the emotional rollercoaster with Joann every single day as time went on.

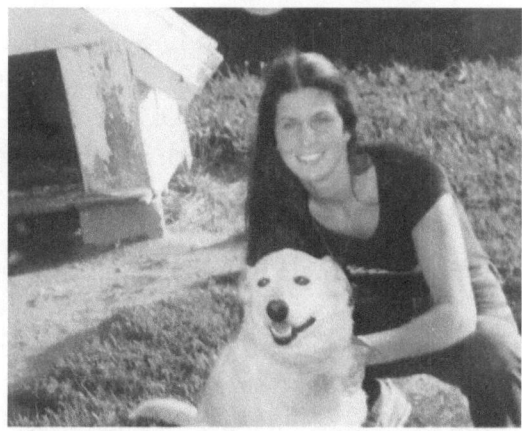

*Lisa Teenager 15*

Lisa was now a high school senior and driving legally! She went to school, held down two and three jobs at a time, had a boyfriend, and was determined to graduate and go to college. Her mother and the antics that she displayed, weighed heavily on her every single day, but Lisa was determined to overcome it all.

Her grandmother was a driving force behind that internal strength. As Lisa was growing up into a young woman, she realized what her grandmother was doing for her; she was supporting Lisa through the madness. Lisa became less angry with the world and more appreciative to have a guiding voice of reason. Rose was a pillar of strength, filled with the wisdom Lisa needed to hear.

Rose was silently compassionate and played hardball like no other. She was strong! Tough as nails! She wanted Lisa to be strong! She silently prayed for Joann to overcome her sickness. This was the internal pain of a mother/grandmother wishing for better but understanding the reality.

The house was filled with so many dysfunctional factors that went way beyond Joann and her illness, which YES, played a huge roll in this mess.

Joann's father was an alcoholic, and he had his own shortcomings and antics that came to light every day as well. He worked very hard but also played hard. There were many disagreements between husband and wife on so many levels. Lisa also took the brunt of her grandfather's ridiculous drunken behaviors and unpredictable anger.

Lisa and her grandfather engaged in many verbal battles, and some became physical. It was the battle of the wills between the two of them, and neither one would back down.

Can you imagine those battles, which mostly seemed to happen around that kitchen table!

## The knights of the round table in constant battle

We all played our parts in this dysfunctional game, with Joann up in the middle of everything. When one battle would break out, it was like a domino effect as we all fought for our place.

Adding to the mix was Joann's youngest brother. He lived there as well, and he had his own internal demons that he was fighting. He had his moments of depression and anger. He also went through a period of intense drug and alcohol use, which further added to this dysfunctional household. He would also bring in his drug infested girlfriends who would stay for short stints.

Just what this household needed more damaged individuals!

It was extremely hard to live there. We co-existed on the eggshells of disaster smashing in those emotional walls on a daily basis. You had to have a tough skin just to survive. Lisa was learning this as she went along. She learned how to internalize everything and remain focused on her mission. The mission at hand was to get out of Dodge as soon as possible.

There were many obstacles to overcome, and the daily grind would become maddening as Joann would feed into this high energy environment as her engines would rev up!

When Joann was feeling extremely manic, she would want to go off on wild adventures. She would take off running, and nobody would know where she was. It was quite difficult to keep up with her when she was in this state of mind. She met many people along the way through her countless hospital stays, emergency room visits, and her mental health office. She knew how to pick out the most dysfunctional people in the mix, and that was who she gravitated to. It was another one of her patterns, and she was like clockwork when she went down this dark path.

Lisa went on many search and rescue missions over the years as Joann would play hide and seek in the seediest parts of town. On more than one occasion, Lisa found herself knee deep in the most dangerous sections of New Haven interacting with homeless people, drunken bums on the streets, and homeless shelters as she was seeking out her lost mother.

Driving through the dark streets of this dangerous town, she would randomly pull over, asking people if they knew her mother. She would even show pictures. When she would mention her mom by name "Joann," there was always a story—and not a pleasant one. Sometimes, Lisa's grandfather would come with her, and they would battle with Joann to come home. She would become loud and aggressive, and they would retreat because of the danger. Joann would always make her way back home somehow, and those were very intense times. Nobody knew exactly what she was doing, and that was scary when you saw the company she kept.

When Joann would finally return home, she would always be a total mess. She would give away all of her money, cigarettes, and even the shoes on her feet, as well as the clothing on her back. Sometimes she would come home wearing other people's clothing that smelled like old fish or the bottom of a dumpster! As she would walk through the door, she looked beaten and worn, feet black from walking barefoot for hours. Sometimes she would have cuts and bruises with no explanation to offer.

She would then retreat to her room and go through the emotional withdrawal of what she put herself through—and the rage would begin. During these times she would end up doing a short stint in the psychiatric unit to regain balance, so to speak. Truly, there was never really any balance. Some moments in time were better than others, and that is the bottom line. That is the ugly truth of mental illness, that insidious beast raging inside Joann's brain every day. This was her battle to fight, and what a difficult one it was.

When Joann would become more balanced, she would display sadness over her continued antics. During these times, her religious side would peak through the clouds and she would spend days weeping, praying, and doing continual rosaries and novenas, begging for forgiveness of all her sins.

*When you think about it, were they really a sin, or the actions of a very sick woman who suffered tremendously?*

Joann would go to church daily during her religious periods. It was during these times that she would walk the fine line of being an angelic angel of God and a sultry seductress of mortal sin, tempting the men of the cloth! As Joann shifted gears so rapidly, what would begin as a cry for help, quickly turned into a sexual battle of a distorted view of attention.

When she set her mind on getting the attention of a priest, she was relentless in her pursuit. She did make a deep connection with a priest at our local church, Father T. In the beginning, you could see he was trying to help her and seemed to be devoted to being her confidant, friend, and mentor. She would speak with him daily and would also go to the rectory for counseling.

Lisa would watch her at times as she would get ready to go to her counseling sessions. She would see the personality transformation right before her eyes. It was mind-blowing to see these events occur. Joann had a ritual, as she lay out her specific clothing on the bed, so meticulous in how she wanted to present herself.

Then the music would come on. She would blast the radio as she did her hair and makeup to perfection. As she smoked away on her cigs (as she called them), she would talk to herself. She had a game plan, and it definitely was not biblical. Her personality would be transformed with every stroke of her mascara. The finishing touch, a brightly colored scarf tied up in her hair. She would put on her chunky wedge heels, and she was ready to go.

Joann always had a certain walk about her when she was presenting this personality, as she would sashay down the hallway, like a movie star making her grand entrance.

As she presented herself to Lisa and her mother, you could even hear the tone in her voice had changed as well.

"Look at me. I look hot right?" Joann boasted.

"Where are you going mom?" Lisa asked, already knowing the answer.

"I am off to see Father T. He loves our sessions," Joann smiled wickedly.

Lisa looked at her, appalled.

"Seriously Mom, he is a priest for Christ sakes! What the hell do you think you are doing?"

"None of your fucking business, you little bitch! You are always judging me. Father T. is a man of God, and he doesn't judge me. He loves me for the sexy woman that I am!" Joann snorted!

"Oh my God, MOM! He doesn't love you! Once again, he is a priest!" Lisa screamed at her over and over again.

"He won't be when I get done with him! Try and stop me Lisa!"

Joann was now laughing and taunting her daughter. Rose stepped up and gave her daughter a few last words before she left the house, but Joann didn't care one bit. She was on a mission, and that was to turn this priest around to the dark side!

This personality of Joann's was too difficult to battle with . . . and they both knew it . . ., so feeling defeated, they both fell into silence. As Joann walked out the door with her car keys in hand, she turned around looked Lisa in the eye, dangling her keys in the air and said, "Catch me if you can!"

You could hear her laughter even after she walked out the door.

Rose turned to Lisa and said, "I am so disgusted. I do not know what I am going to do with that girl."

"There is nothing you can do grandma. She is sick and refuses our help. How can we battle this illness? It is too big for all of us combined," Lisa's voice sounded annoyed and broken at the same time.

"Let's just hope Father T. is stronger than she is." Rose said with a bit of hopefulness in her voice.

"Don't count on it," Lisa replied.

*\*\*\*After countless sessions with Joann and a budding friendship that had many tongues wagging in the church, Father T. stepped down as a priest and moved to Vermont with another woman. Joann stayed in contact with him for many years even after he was a married man.*

# Chapter 15

# Transitions

As time moved forward and they were all co-existing in that house on the hill, so much transpired daily. Every single day was a "hold on to the seat of your pants" type of day. You never knew what was going to come at you next.

*Imagine living this type of lifestyle as you were trying to grow up into a mature, confident, and productive adult!*

Could someone actually walk away from this mess unscathed by the rituals of this unhealthy environment?

That answer would be a big NO!

There were many transitions along the way, and Joann kept on coming out swinging. There was always a new friend, a new drama, and a new plan. The cycle was endless, and nobody could keep up with this manic pace.

Lisa went on to finish off her senior year of high school, and graduated with honors. This was a very proud moment for her because the path that she has traveled was one hell of a ride, but she made it.

## Graduation Day

Standing among her peers, she was looking around feeling a sense of accomplishment.

Lisa was also sad for many reasons. The sadness came from the fact that as she looked around, she was very well aware that nobody truly knew her or what she had been through. All of these young men and women were ready to celebrate and move on to the next stages of their lives never knowing what happened to that little girl who lived in "the house of horrors."

As Lisa pushed that thought out of her head, another one came forward. I wished my grandmother was here to listen to my name being called! She did not come to the graduation because of her blindness. She was not comfortable in big crowds.

As teachers and delegates got up to speak one by one, Lisa heard the words of her grandmother who waiting at home for her.

"Lisa I am so proud of you, and I always knew you would make it. I love you." said Rose as Lisa made her way out the door with her cap and gown in hand.

Lisa stopped for a moment feeling quite emotional at the words she just heard.

Now, looking back at her grandmother sitting in the chair at that "famous" kitchen table, she simply said, "I love you too."

As the next image popped in her head as she sat there, there was her mom. She was there in the stands with a few of her family members, and Lisa prayed that she would be "good" just for one day. She was silently begging God to not let her mom embarrass her. Lisa's fingers were crossed so tight that they left red marks on them.

Lastly, the gears shift to her dad.

Just before the ceremony started, Lisa stood alone nervously waiting for him to arrive. Would he show up? Would he miss her big moment?

John never liked to be anywhere close to Joann because it was always an explosive scene.

Just as Lisa was giving up hope, here he came, walking up larger than life! Lisa ran to him, threw her arms around him, and hugged him tight.

"You came, you came!" she squealed.

"Of course, I came. I would never miss my baby graduate high school. I am so proud of you," said John. "Now go get in line with your friends and always know that I love you."

"Thank you, daddy. I love you too," Lisa said as she kissed his cheek, and off she went. As she turned around for one last look, there was her dad standing there with his own mother and sister. Lisa felt so very proud.

Just as quickly as the ceremony started, it was over! All of the students threw their caps in the air and cheered wildly.

The Class of 1983, West Haven High School, made it. We were done with our high school years, and now it was on to new adventures.

Lisa was a deep thinker, and as she looked around, she knew that she would never see many of these people ever again, but that meant hopefully, new beginnings.

**Transitions**

Would Joann allow her daughter to grow successfully?

Lisa was accepted into a business school for a Secretarial Program. Lisa's true love was art, and her biggest dream was to go to art school. However, because of money and circumstances, she had to put that dream aside and be more practical about her decision making. She knew she needed to have a career that would come quickly so she could make enough money to take care of herself and move out. That was the main goal.

When Lisa announced that she was going to start business school directly out of high school (it was a two-year course condensed into a year), Joann put up a big fuss. She did not want her daughter attending school—or leaving the house for that matter! Joann figured once Lisa was done with high school, she would stay home and take care of her.

Another distorted scenario inside the mind of a sick woman.

This was the last thing on Lisa's mind. She had taken care of her mother her whole life, and that was not her goal for the future. The conversation about Lisa furthering her education was a high-fueled battle of the wills. Lisa had Rose on her side which was helpful, but it was a bloody battle to the finish.

## The College Conversation

It was the end of May 1983, and Lisa received her acceptance letter to The Stone Business School, in New Haven, Connecticut. When Lisa opened that envelope, there was a huge sense of pride as she read the word, "Accepted." This word meant so much to her. It was exciting to see her hard work and determination had paid off, but for Lisa that word meant so much more. It meant that she would finally find her place, and this would allow her an opportunity to move forward with her life. It was a place of community, goals, and belonging. A chance to finally be free!

Lisa walked into the kitchen because she wanted to share the news with her grandmother and uncle. They were sitting at the kitchen table chatting, as Lisa let out a big squeal of excitement!

"Guess what! Guess what! I was accepted to the business school I applied to! I am going to college!" Lisa was standing there feeling such a sense of accomplishment, but before her grandmother or uncle could reply, she felt deep breathing on the back of her neck as her mother ran up behind her.

Lisa jumped as her mom yelled, "The hell you are! You are going to stay here and take care of me. You owe me!"

Lisa whipped around and screamed back into her mother's face.

"I owe you nothing! I have spent my whole life taking care of you, and it is my turn now!" Lisa was then met with a strong hand across her face, as she felt the burn sting her cheek.

Her uncle got up and jumped in between mother and daughter, as Rose began to scream at them to knock it off immediately.

"Michael, stop her, stop her! Where is Lisa?"

"I am here grandma. I am coming to you!" Lisa grabbed her hand and held it tight, as her uncle wrestled with Joann until she calmed down.

"Knock it the fuck off. What the hell is wrong with you?"

"Lisa deserves to go to college," Rose chimed in, with a stern tone. "Joann, Lisa does not need to take care of you. She needs her education. You need to stop this at once."

Lisa felt strong standing next to her grandmother, because she knew that her mother, as much as she yelled, would not go against her own mother. She also felt a sense of protection having her uncle there to back her up!

"Lisa has a full life ahead of her, and she deserves to do the things that she wants to. I am proud of her, and you should be too," Rose stated.

"Oh yeah, that is right, whatever 'Mona Lisa' wants, 'Mona Lisa' gets. Spoiled little bitch. She deserves nothing. I am the one who deserves everything!" Joann snorted angrily.

As her brother Michael rolled his eyes, he blatantly told her to shut up! Joann turned her anger back to him, calling him a no-good mother fucker and a turn coat. He glared at her with such contempt and anger but decided to remain quiet. You could see the steam coming from his ears!

Rose raised her voice and stated there would be no more arguing and this conversation was over.

"Lisa will attend college. Deal with it, Joann."

Joann replied, "Oh don't you worry, I will deal with it, my way!" She stomped out the door cursing and swearing.

Lisa sat down next to her grandmother and uncle. They all just took a moment of silence as her mother was mentally draining on all of them. Michael looked over at Lisa and said, "I'm proud of you kid!"

Lisa smiled at him and gave him a big hug. Rose also stated the same thing, as she let out a big sigh.

"I do not know what we are going to do with your mother. She is completely out of control." .Rose stated.

"I don't know either Grandma. She is going to continue to give me a hard time," Lisa replied.

"We will figure it out as we go," said Rose.

With graduation behind her, Lisa focused her energy on preparing for college. She only had a two-week window off before the program began. While many of her friends were enjoying their last summer of freedom, Lisa was hitting the books.

Party time was over, and a seriousness came over her. She knew she had to be successful. She knew she had to prove her mother wrong. As Lisa was getting all of her last-minute details taken care of before her first day of school, she got into an automobile accident. Her car was totaled. She was banged up, but okay.

This incident fueled Joann's unrealistic ideas that her daughter was meant to stay home with her.

"This is a sign," Joann told Lisa. "You see, you go against me and God—this is what happens to you! Next time you will surely die. You cannot leave the house anymore unless it is with me!"

"OH MY GOD, MOM, stop it! You are crazy, and I am not staying home with you! I will find a way!"

Joann kept on taunting her until her mother chimed in and stated that Lisa would take the city bus to school. With or without a car, she was going.

Joann got up and screamed in Lisa's face.

"You are going to die. Do you hear me. You have been warned!" Joann was waving her finger in her face.

Lisa could hear her harrowing voice echo through her head over and over again, "YOU HAVE BEEN WARNED!"

Lisa felt defeated in this moment. She did not have any support from her own mother, her vehicle was totaled, and now she would be forced to take the city bus through the worst sections of New Haven, just to get an education.

She thought, *Is it even worth it, maybe my mother is right, I do not deserve anything.*

An over-whelming sense of sadness came over her as she wanted her mother to be proud of her.

*Why does every conversation always have to end in a battle of the wills, with me always feeling guilty? It is not fair.*

As Lisa looked over to see her grandmother sitting there sipping her coffee peacefully, she said to herself, "I have to do this for myself. My grandmother believes in me, and I want to make her proud of all of the things that I am trying to do."

Unfortunately, Lisa and her grandmother also traveled a turbulent road for a long time, because of her deep-seated pain and anger from her past. Lisa took a lot of those dark feelings out on her. She lashed out at her grandmother frequently, but Rose always remained extremely strong, taking each lashing with courage and wisdom. She remained supportive no matter how difficult it became for her. Lisa felt bad thinking about how hard she had been on this woman who had loved her so deeply.

She sighed thinking, "I need to be like my Grandma Rose. I need to be tough! It is time to stand up and fight for me. Nothing is going to stop me, especially *Hurricane Joann*!

# Chapter 16

# Growing Up In Spite of Joann

Time moved forward, and Lisa attended school with many difficulties along the way. Joann made it quite difficult for her and tried to sabotage her journey. During this time period, Joann continued to struggle with her mental illness, once again taking herself off of her medications because she was magically "CURED."

Then the downward spiral began.

Lisa thought to herself, "This could not be worse timing!"

Every single day was a battle, if not with words, with fists, or her mother purposely destroying anything related to Lisa's school work. For a year and a half, Lisa got up every morning at 5 a.m., had her coffee and breakfast with her grandparents, and prepared herself for the day ahead. Lisa's days were hard and long. She would catch the 6:30 a.m. bus to school at the bottom of the hill in all types of weather. She would be in school all day and then start her homework on the bus ride home. Lisa had a system, and she was sticking by it.

Once she was home, she would continue to do her homework, grab something to eat, and get ready for work. Lisa worked four nights a week and all-day Saturday. Because she did not have a vehicle, she would try to get a ride with someone if she could, or she was forced to walk. Sometimes, her mother would give her a ride, but that was the last person she wanted to ask. If she asked for help from her mom, it always came with a price tag.

Joann was riding the highs and lows without her medications, and she would constantly unleash her vile behaviors onto the whole family. The last thing Lisa wanted to do was to get in a car with her because she drove like a maniac. Sometimes she would allow Lisa to drive, but most of the time she liked to scare the shit out of her, by flying down the roads barely stopping for red lights or traffic.

"Hold on tight Lisa, maybe I will crash into that car in front of us, and we will both die together. This way you will never be able to leave me!" Joann would sometimes scream.

Lisa would hold on for dear life, screaming at her mother to stop driving so insanely, but Joann never listened. When Joann would finally come to a halt, Lisa would jump out of the car getting away from her as fast as she could. Joann could be heard laughing wildly, as she would speed off in a cloud of smoke! Lisa lived in a constant world of extreme madness, under the demented thumb of her twisted mother.

At night when Lisa would finally return home from work exhausted, it was always back to the books.

One night as Lisa was going through her back pack, looking for her homework sheets, she was puzzled because she could not find them.

"Grandma, has anyone been in my back pack today?" she asked.

"Lisa, where was your backpack?" Rose questioned.

"It was on the chair in the corner. I left it there so I could finish it tonight, as it is due tomorrow."

"I think your mother was over there earlier. Go ask her if she saw it."

An instant wave of fear and anger washed over Lisa's face at the same time. She was exhausted, stressed out, and wanted to go to sleep. She had no time for games.

"Mom, Mom, have you seen my homework?"

Joann came waltzing into the kitchen with a cheeky look on her face. She held up the homework and said, "Are you looking for this?" Then she proceeded to light it on fire with her lighter. Lisa lunged forward frantically grabbing the papers. She burned her hand as she tried to put it out. Joann's sick laughter grew louder as Lisa's head began to spin.

"What the fuck is wrong with you? Why would you do such a thing? You mean spirited bitch!"

Joann's laughter turned into anger as she unleashed her fury onto her.

"I told you, No School!, No School! Do you hear me?" Joann was screaming with wild untamed energy! "Those papers are evil, and they were calling out to me tonight, telling me to burn them all! I am saving you from the devil!" Then Joann broke down into tears, sobbing uncontrollably. "Nobody understands me!"

Because of all of this commotion, everyone congregated into the kitchen. Lisa's grandparents, and her uncle were now trying to calm Joann down and console her after this horrible display. Once they were able to finally calm her down, Rose instructed her husband and son to escort her to her bedroom to lay down. She cried herself to sleep that night. She was weeping about so many things. The loss of her son and her destroyed marriage. The loss of her daughter who was growing up right before her eyes, and not wanting to face the fact that she could not control her any longer.

Joann wept for every piece of her life that had brought her to this very moment. As the song, "Sad Eyes" played on her little transiter radio, she finally fell asleep.

Everyone went back to what they were doing, so they could regroup and take space for a moment. Nobody, said a single word. Here it was, more silence to endure.

Lisa stood there in the kitchen, feeling totally distraught. As she held those burned papers in her hands, she allowed a few tears to flow. She was shaking. Then she heard a voice behind her.

"Lisa are you still there, are you ok?"

Lisa wiped her face and turned around. "Yes, grandma I am here. I am going to sit at the table and do my homework."

"Ok, I will sit with you. There is coffee on the stove if you want some," Rose offered.

Suddenly, her grandfather appeared back into the kitchen looking sadly at his granddaughter.

"Sit down and get started. I will pour you a cup of coffee," he said.

Next Michael walked into the kitchen. He quietly grabbed a cup of coffee and sat with the three of them. Nobody said a word, as Lisa worked feverishly trying to put all of her papers back together. As she was re-writing all of her work, focusing on trying to figure out what her mother burned, she could feel all of her family members silently supporting her. She thought to herself, "They were rooting for me to succeed." She knew what she had to do, and succeeding was the only answer. When Lisa was done with everything, she took a long hot shower and laid down on the couch. She set her alarm for 5 a.m. and grimaced at the thought of it.

Just as quickly as she closed her eyes, she heard the alarm blaring in her ears. Lisa instantly jumped up and was moving quickly. A new day began. She took a deep breath and whispered out loud, "You Can Do This."

Lisa had to dress in business attire every day for school. Her mother secretly put cigarette holes in one of her brand-new blouses. As Lisa reached for this blouse in the closet, she was mortified to see that it was destroyed in such a devious way. That was it, she had had enough! Lisa worked hard for her money, and she needed to look the part for the business school. Her mother was destroying everything that she was trying to accomplish.

The last straw came when Joann burned Lisa's clothing.

It was time for a huge battle, and Lisa did not care anymore—she was done.

## The Battle and The Hospital Stay—Here we go again

As she got dressed for school that morning, she remained calm. Lisa tucked the charred blouse in the back of her closet and prepared for the day. She knew her mother was waiting for an explosive response. She wanted the instant battle, and on that day, Lisa decided she wasn't going to give it to her, just yet!

She had a game plan, and she was not going to allow her mother to ruin her school day. It was coming to the end of her program, and Lisa could not afford to miss a thing. She was working extremely hard to pass with honors. It was a goal that she set for herself, and she intended to see it through.

As Lisa walked into the kitchen, her mother was there waiting with bated breath. Lisa tried to ignore her as she was getting her backpack together so she could make her way to the bus stop.

"Lisa, why are you not wearing that beautiful white blouse today; you know, the new one that you just bought?"

Lisa was fuming on the inside as Joann just pushed every button with one sentence! Joann was so good at pushing buttons, and she knew how to go directly for the jugular. One could say that she was a seasoned professional.

"I couldn't find it in my closet MOM, so I decided to go with the pink one; you know, YOUR favorite color!" Lisa was glaring at her with a half-smile, as Joann glared back. "I am on my way out now, but we will definitely talk after school."

Lisa looked over at her grandmother and said goodbye for the day. As she stepped out the door, she took in a deep breath of fresh air.

*You can do this Lisa. Put it all aside until you get home, focus.*

She went about her day, blocking out all that was happening, and what she needed to do when she returned home. Lisa was accomplishing great things in school, and it felt fantastic. She always knew that she was smart, but her past trauma damaged her in so many ways. Learning did not come easy for Lisa because all of the past abuse and trauma that clouded her mind. She was always battling herself inside her thoughts and fears, so that she could remain clear and focused. It was a daunting task to be in battle with yourself every single day, so that you could become successful.

*Remember . . . Nobody ever walks away from trauma or abuse unscathed—there is always a scar that remains:*
*Developmental Disabilities – PTSD – Memory Blocks – Blank Spaces.*

When the day was over, Lisa made her long trek back home. When she stepped off of the bus, she was flooded with every thought, feeling, and emotion that she had packed away from that morning. As she made her way ever so slowly up the big hill, a warm breeze was hitting her face. With each and every step, she was emotionally unpacking all of the baggage that she had suppressed. She was completely dreading what would come next—the battle!

Lisa was trying to plan out what she was going to say, and how she was going to approach it all. She knew her mother was always a "loose cannon," so to speak, and you never knew what level of nastiness you were going to get. Deep inside her soul, she already knew how it was going to end, but she tried to be slightly optimistic. Lisa believed this was her own way of protecting her brain from further trauma. As she hit the top of the hill, she stood there for a few minutes before she crossed the busy street. Lisa watched the cars whiz on by for a few moments as she was mentally preparing herself just to cross the road. Finally, she just did it. As she made her way up the dirt driveway, she was dragging her feet.

When Lisa hit the front door and opened it, she was instantly greeted with fury.

**The Battle**

"You fucking liar! You little whore!" Joann was screaming.

"What the hell is wrong with you?" Lisa screamed back!

Joann pulled out the blouse from behind her back and threw it at Lisa.

"I found this in the back of your closet, where you stashed it bitch!" Joann snorted.

Lisa marched right on by her, dropping her bags on the chair, and turned in a fury of anger like she had never felt before.

"YOU NASTY SELF-CENTERED BITCH OF A MOTHER!" How dare you wreck my clothing! How dare you continue to try to wreck my life! I am done with your bullshit! DONE—DONE—DONE—DO YOU HEAR ME!"

"Lisa, what is going on now?" Rose chimed in,

"Grandma, this bitch burned my brand-new blouse with cigarette holes and put it back in my closet, and she is twisted enough to think I was going to wear it! She is an evil witch, and I hate her!"

Before Lisa could say anything else, Joann came charging at her like a raging bull, full steam ahead, grabbing her and slamming her to the floor. Total chaos broke out as Joann continued to attack Lisa.

Rose was screaming for her husband, and he came running in from the other room pulling Joann off of her.

Rose continued to scream "Everyone Stop! I mean it—Everyone Stop!"

Lisa's grandfather held onto Joann tight, as she got back up on her feet. As she wiped her lip, blood trickled down her mouth, which fueled her anger even more.

"I wish you were dead! Do you hear me dead! I never hated anyone in my entire life as much as I hate you!" Lisa stood there staring her mother in the face, challenging her to come at her again, but to her surprise, Joann just started to cry.

Then she took it to the next level and became completely hysterical. Joann ran violently into the bedroom as she proceeded to throw everything around the room, breaking several items. She was screaming at top of her lungs, cursing at God and the whole family. There was no consoling her or taming the beast within.

As Lisa and her grandparents stood in the kitchen, there was nothing they could do but allow her to rage on until her fury was finally over. When everything went quiet and the dust settled, the room was completely destroyed. (Lisa's items included because they were forced to share a room). Joann once again classically dropped onto the bed and silently sobbed.

Rose called her other daughter and explained what had happened and asked her to call the doctor. Joann needed to go back to the hospital. This was always a difficult thing for everyone to endure, Joann included. We had traveled down this road countless times before, and it always ended up the same way. We had the rise and the fall, followed by the hospital stay.

Mental illness is a cruel beast that not only swallows up the person who is ill, but everyone that surrounds them. The one's closest, hurt the most. You may think that the hospital stay was a big victory, but truthfully it was not. It was just another stay that Joann would hold against her daughter and family for life.

Another stay that would include Joann fighting everyone, further hurting herself along the way. In her mind, it was like being locked in jail and being punished for an illness that she never asked for. She was not wrong! Joann held on tight to that anger and used it as a "guilt trip" whenever it worked in her favor.

The only win here, was that Lisa could finish school in peace, and Joann would be safe. So, if you want to call it a win-win—go ahead—but the raw truth is that nobody is winning when it comes to a broken heart.

Joann left that day going to the hospital for a twenty day stay. This was just long enough for Lisa to finish out her classes. (Sometimes God steps in to give a helping hand).

When Joann returned home, she had to face the reality. Lisa was growing up and graduating from The Stone School of Business, completing what she started. Joann had to face it. She has lost control of her little girl. Her little girl was now a woman.

*What will Joann do to get it all back?*

# Chapter 17

# Not A Child Anymore—
# Time in a Bottle . . .

After graduation day, life changed in many ways. First of all, Lisa graduated with honors like she had promised herself. Joann was able to come to the graduation with her brother and father by her side. Lisa moved forward with her first "grown up" job, and bought herself a new vehicle.

Life was starting to move quickly, and Lisa was embracing every single change as it presented itself. Her uncle finally made his own step out into the world and moved out of the house.

**Then there were four!**

Joann continued to ride that mental health roller-coaster as the weeks and months moved on. She was trying to accept the fact that her daughter was growing up and making her own decisions. This was very hard for her, as she never wanted her daughter to leave her. The thought of this brought up every feeling of loss that one could imagine. Joann lost her only son, and her husband moved forward with his life. She continued to battle her inner demons fighting tooth and nail to keep them at bay.

At times she managed to hold herself together for a little while, when she was taking care of herself. Joann would go in waves. When she was being proactive, going to therapy and taking her medications, she would settle down for a bit. She and Lisa would actually have decent conversations together. Joann would try so hard to connect with Lisa. Deep down inside she knew the damage that was caused, and she truly felt such pride at Lisa's accomplishments, in spite of all that had transpired.

The down fall was Lisa and Joann were still forced to share a room together, and this was unacceptable to Lisa. She felt stuck and trapped in her past. She fought so desperately to get away from it, but every time she walked into her own bedroom, it was like a huge punch in the stomach. Here was the reality. Lisa could not afford to be out on her own yet, and she had to continue to work hard to get out! That was always her game plan—Get Out!

There were continual battles over a smoke-filled bedroom, blaring music, and bed wetting (Joann would frequently wet the bed). Lisa had been on the latter end of that nightmare far too many times, and the damage ran deep.

Lisa slept on the couch or reclining chair more than she slept in her own room. It was very hard to co-exist in such a way. She knew her grandparents had done the best that they could for her, but it was not the lifestyle she wanted. She couldn't do it anymore. The years of trauma and abuse wore her down in so many ways. Everything she had ever accomplished had to come with a huge battle attached to it, and she was tired.

Lisa and Joann rode that roller-coaster together for years, and Lisa wanted off. She was going to do everything in her power to move forward and live her "own" life.

Joann, on the other hand, had her own plan. Joann always envisioned her and Lisa living together forever. Lisa would take care of Joann for the rest of her life. In Joann's mind, Lisa owed her—and owed her big time. This was a huge delusional fantasy that she carried for years! This is why she would try to sabotage everything Lisa did, because she knew that eventually she would leave. That was not in Joann's game plan, so she was relentless and calculating every step of the way.

The one thing Joann could not do was to stop time. Time was

moving on, and Lisa was gaining ground. She changed jobs, landing the job that she wanted, working for Miles Pharmaceuticals as a medical secretary for a research team. This was another goal that she set for herself and achieved. On the day of the interview, Joann created a huge fuss at home, shaking Lisa to the core. They battled fiercely that morning, which left them both in tears. Lisa had to find a way to pull herself together before she walked out the door. This was the pattern, one step forward, two steps backward as Joann fought her every step of the way.

When Lisa was put into these situations, she would suck it all up internally, put on her game face, and forge into battle. The battle of the wills! Lisa was also doing the same thing as her mother she was battling herself daily.

Oh the patterns—those self-taught dysfunctional coping skills that we learn over the years to survive trauma and abuse. Along the way, Joann inadvertently taught her daughter the same skills that she engaged in for years, even before Lisa was born. Now these awful traits had been bestowed upon Lisa like a "mental curse."

The battles surrounded her like war torn country. That is what she felt like every single day. The dysfunction raged on like wild fire. Everyone in the house on the hill battled the flames of Joann.

As for Joann, she rode the waves of emotion, fighting each season as it was presented before her. The highs, the lows, and the mania. She was classic with her behaviors which mirrored the time of year. Every season had a different Joann, and her family would prepare for all the twists and turns. It was mentally and emotionally draining.

As the storm brewed, everyone felt the uneasy energy walking on egg shells, as not to set off the beast within. They all silently waited, as they knew it was coming. Joann would prime up slowly, and then with the flip of a switch, it was game on! The storm would explode, and Joann would be out of control like a tornado sucking up everything in her path, tearing it up until there was nothing left. She was brutal with her tongue and violent with her fists. In these moments of mania, she felt larger than life, as if nothing could touch her, but like all big storms, they eventually crash. As the tornado of Joann would come crashing to the ground, so did she.

That is when the deep depression would set in and the tears would flow like the River Jordan. During these dark times, there was no consoling her. She had to ride it out like she was programed to do so, and you could not break the pattern.

It was heart-breaking to watch, and it never got any easier to witness as the years carried on. This was the lifestyle we were all living. It was not just Joann who was suffering, but her family as well.

Imagine her parents, not really knowing what else to do to help their daughter. They had been at it for years! They sent her out into the world with high hopes, only to have her return even more damaged than when she left. Pat struggled with his drinking problem, and Rose was blind. Not only did they have to deal with a daughter who was mentally ill, but a granddaughter who was angry with the world, damaged so profusely by the trauma. Pat and Rose struggled tremendously trying to keep the household intact, and they did the best that they could.

As for Lisa, imagine having to share a room with the person who had hurt her so much. She was living with guilt over the fact that she felt hate in her heart for her own mother, but she also knew that her love was deeper. Another internal battle.

Every day she would walk out that door, whether it was to go to school or work, and she would internalized everything, just to survive. Inside her mind, body, and soul, this terror raged on, and she had to bury it all so deep. Lisa would pray every night that this pain would never see the light of day. This was the only way that she knew she could survive it all. She had to remain silent, so she could live. Imagine how she suffered alone. Imagine what great strength and strong will it took to keep pushing forward. She was driven by it!

Another lesson Lisa learned along the way was to never give up. She learned that also from Joann. Joann could have given up countless times, because she traveled at the lowest of the lows far too many times for anyone to count, but she always got back up swinging. Her will to live and survive was surreal. Lisa would never admit to it, but she knew where that inner drive came from, and how it was embedded into her.

When the time came for Lisa to finally claim her freedom, it came in the most surprising way.

Lisa met a man named John. It was unexpected and a true blessing. She fell in love with him immediately, and he said it was love at first sight. They were soulmates, that was undeniable. This beautiful gift was the final stepping stone Lisa needed to take that leap of faith.

All the years of suffering, fighting, and enduring got her to this place right here. She had met the man of her dreams, and they were going to get married. It was all happening so quickly. Not only were they going to be married, but they were moving from Connecticut to Massachusetts. Lisa loved the country and the beauty of nature. It was always her passion to be in the trees. That beautiful smell of those tall pine trees were so enticing as they called her name.

Then the unthinkable happened.

Lisa's Grandmother Rose passed away suddenly from a massive heart attack. Everyone was devastated, and Lisa's heart broke because she wanted her grandmother to be a part of her wedding day. She thought about how her grandmother would "feel her dress on her." When Lisa went to the prom, her grandmother felt her dress and was able to describe it completely.

Rose said to Lisa, "One day I will do this with your wedding dress!"

Those words were ringing in her ears on the day they buried her.

As Lisa stood alongside her family, she whispered silently, "I know you will walk down the aisle with me. I love you so much."

Of course, Joann was destroyed after losing her mom. She loved her mother so very much. It may not have seemed that way, but mental illness draws out a darkness that masks the true person. Joann loved her mother intensely and completely, and for her to pass away, it was way more than she could bear. That thought of losing someone else in her life put her completely over the top.

After Rose's funeral, Joann told Lisa plans had to change.

"You cannot leave me ever! Do you hear me Lisa—It is you and me always—Got it?"

Lisa's heart was ever more conflicted. She knew what she wanted and had to figure out how she was going to get there.

JOANN . . . was a huge obstacle that stood in her way of happiness and freedom.

# Chapter 18

# A Battle For Freedom

After the passing of Rose, the house had a certain emptiness about it that was daunting. Rose was the center of the universe in the house on the hill. Her empty chair at the kitchen table said it all. Joann went into a deep state of depression. She would lay on her mother's bed and just sob. She would look up on the wall at the picture of Jesus, and she would curse him for taking her mother away from her.

There was no consoling her as she lay there day after day, grieving to the deepest of levels. The hardest part for Joann was that life still went on, and she was angry with all of us for doing so. She would curse us for living or laughing. She would go over the last moments of Rose's life in her head, and she would repeat those words over and over again out loud for all of us to hear.

Joann did not know what to do. She had always turned to her mother for support and advice. Now all she was left with was her mother's bathrobe and her memories to comfort her. She would hold that robe up to her nose and smell the essence of her mom, and the tears would flow. It truly was a sad time for all of us, but when you added in the deep emotions drawn forward by her mental illness, those feelings were intensified a thousand times over.

During this time of great mourning, Joann didn't realize that Lisa was making her plans to leave. Lisa was talking to other family members, and of course her fiancé, about her plans, but Joann was left out of these serious conversations. This was a time of transitions in many ways.

Two weeks after the death of Rose, John moved to Massachusetts to take on a new job. Lisa would visit him on the weekends. This was very difficult for Lisa to be without him after the loss of her grandmother, and she would count each day until the weekends would arrive. She engrossed herself in her work, working out, and spending time with her dog.

Lisa felt like she was running again. This was a feeling she did not want to have any more in her life, but she couldn't seem to outrun it.

*Run, Lisa, Run*, were the words that she would hear in her head over and over.

When she was home with her mother and grandfather, she would tread lightly so as to not rock the boat. During those long walks alone on the beach with her dog Champ, she thought long and hard about how she was going to break the news to her mother that she was leaving. It was going to be a reality that Joann was going to have to face. Lisa dreaded the thought of what this conversation would look and sound like. The anxiety would feel so overwhelming that she would shake from the inside out. The only peace and comfort that she could find was being at the beach with her dog, sitting in the sand and just being in the moment. With her trusty companion by her side, she would close her eyes and allow the soft wind to blow through her hair as the smell of the salt air ran right through her soul. As the sound of the waves came crashing to the shore, it was like being rocked as a baby.

In those brief moments, Lisa felt completely free, and it was heavenly. It is amazing that some of the coping skills that we learn as children can effectively carry over into our adult lives.

Lisa knew what she had to do, and that was to drop the proverbial bomb. Oh the anguish that she felt, because as much as she wanted her freedom, she didn't want to hurt her mom. Lisa knew how Joann felt about loss. They lived it together, mother and daughter, side by side. Lisa was dragged down a path that she never deserved, but at the same time, she knew deep in her heart that she was supposed to be there for her mother. Lisa lived the nightmare with Joann and felt every blow along the way. She knew by telling her mother that she was leaving would have the same effect on her like the day she lost her son and now her own mother.

Lisa did not want to be that person in her mother's life to hurt her in such a way, but she knew it would be the only way she could have a chance at happiness. The thought of freedom rang in her ears, as the darkness continued to poke at her heart—oh, the conflict ran deeper than words could ever say.

Lisa had made her choice and it was time.

## The Conversation

The day had come, and Lisa would have the conversation that would change her and Joann's life forever. She knew she had to do it alone, so she told her fiancé John she would handle it. He was worried about her as he learned fairly quickly the highs and lows of Joann. They had not been together very long before John met with the wrath of Joann on a few occasions.

Did he have cause to be worried? The answer was *YES*.

Lisa forewarned her grandfather ahead of time that she was going to have this conversation, and he looked at her and just groaned with a deep sigh. She said to him, "Grandpa it is time." He wished her luck and retreated to his bedroom.

Joann was sitting at the kitchen table in her mother's chair. Since Rose's passing, Joann claimed that spot for herself, and nobody was going to argue with her. Her mood was foul most of the time, and she would talk to herself all of the time.

Lisa walked into the kitchen with her nerves tingling in every inch of her body. She stood there in the hallway for a moment mentally preparing herself for this inevitable conversation. She then took a deep breath walked forward .

"Mom, I need to talk to you about something."

Joann turned her head towards Lisa and said, "YAAAAA." with a glare. It was like she knew what was coming.

Lisa wanted to turn around and run, but she stood there calmly.

"Mom, you know John and I want to be married right?"

Again, Joann snarled, "YAAAAA LISA."

"Well, we have decided that we will be married in November, and I will be moving with him to Massachusetts in September." Lisa just stood there and waited for the explosion.

Joann just stared at Lisa for a few minutes not saying a word. This worried her more than an explosion. Lisa was internally shaking as Joann eyed her up in down with such contempt in her eyes and then BOOM!

"What the fuck are you talking about you little bitch whore! Do you want me to fuck you up right now! Are you out of your mind thinking you can leave me!"

Lisa tried to interject, but Joann was on a roll and she exploded to the highest extent. Lisa's grandfather came running in the room with the dog in tow.

"Joann, Joann, calm down! Do you hear me? Lisa has the right to live her life, and this is something you know your mother would want for her. Be happy for her."

Joann stopped dead in her tracks, got up, and ran out of the room hysterically crying and screaming, "God why are you so cruel to me, taking away everyone that I love! I thought you were my friend Jesus Christ." Joann dropped to the bed and sobbed uncontrollably. She was lost in her own heartache and sorrow. She could not see beyond it; she was buried in it.

As Lisa and her grandfather sat in the kitchen talking, they could hear the continual cries of Joann. It was actually heartbreaking to listen to her.

After a long period of time, Joann emerged from the bedroom, looking battered and broken. She sat down next to Lisa.

"OK you win. I hope you are happy that you are killing your mother. I hope you will be happy moving away, knowing every single day that you hurt your own mother more than anyone else ever could. Go be happy Lisa because you are a selfish girl."

Lisa took in every single word as she burned inside. Those words, those hideous words would scar her soul forever, bringing continued guilt bestowed upon her like a curse. Lisa would have to carry this with her, but the thoughts of being with John and finding happiness outweighed those nasty words. Lisa looked at her mother square in the eyes.

"Mom, I am not a girl, I am a woman. I love you, and I will always love you, but it is my time to live. I will always be here for you, but it is time that I move forward. This is my decision, and I hope you can be happy for John and me. We love each other so much. Be excited there is a wedding in the future, and you are the mother of the bride."

Wow, Lisa surprised herself with the words of wisdom that just came out of her mouth. It was like her grandmother was whispering in her ear. Lisa felt a moment of pride and empowerment. She was not backing down, and she felt her spirit move her in that direction—forward.

Joann looked at her daughter, and the pain on her face was evident.

Lisa felt it, her grandfather felt it. Lisa got up and hugged her mother. Joann sobbed in her arms. All Lisa could do was hold her tight. The thoughts of the past came rushing through her mind like a fast-moving picture show. Every memory good and bad flew by, and Lisa felt dizzy. As Joann continued to cry, Lisa just held on tight until it was over. It was like a freight train of emotions came barreling through the house, and all she could do was hold on.

When the sobbing stopped, Lisa wiped away her mother's tears and said, "Mom, you will always have me. It will be ok."

"Ok Lisa," Joann responded. She got up and went back to her room. Joann had moved into her mother's room claiming that as her own as well. It was her comfort zone. Joann retreated there for the rest of the night.

Lisa went outside and sat on the back steps with her dog. She looked up at the sky, and the stars seemed to shine brighter than ever. She looked up and said, "Thank you grandma." Then Lisa's mind wandered to her brother, her guardian angel. She always felt him close by. As kids they loved looking at the stars together. "Jon Jon, I know you are there. Please know that I love and miss you so much. I wish you were here with me."

As a few tears dripped from her eyes, Champ leaned in close as if to say *I am here with you.*

She hugged him tightly and said, "Get ready for new adventures, because you are coming with me."

After that night, time moved quickly. Lisa was busy working, preparing for the wedding, and her impending move. Joann would have her ups and downs over the next few months. There were moments when she seemed happy for Lisa, but with the flip of a switch, her negative badgering would emerge.

Lisa rode this complex rollercoaster of transition with Joann, and it was one hell of a ride. The bumps and bruises were quite painful, and the damage was running deep.

Joann was so unpredictable, and she switched gears so quickly it was always hard to keep up. Just when you thought you may be ahead of the game, she would push you ten steps back!

Over the next few months, many things happened for Lisa. She left the job that she loved to be with the man that she loved. She moved to Massachusetts, and they bought their first home together. Lisa started a new job and was trying to adjust to a brand-new life with the love of her life by her side, and her faithful dog Champ.

So many transitions. The biggest one was not seeing, or being with her mother every single day. Not having to share the same room with her, have the same fights with her daily, and not being subjected to her abuse. It was a lot to take in.

Of course, Joann did not remain quiet. Her new tool and weapon of choice was the telephone. Joann called Lisa daily and not just once a day, many times the calls would exceed six to ten calls.

Lisa's only defense was the answering machine. When she was not up for handling another battle, she let the machine do it!

## On November 29, 1986—John and Lisa were married.
## Mr. & Mrs. John Zarcone

It was a cold but beautiful day. The sun was shining as they entered the church, but as they were leaving, it began to snow. John and Lisa felt it was a sign of renewal and happiness to come.

It was a very emotional day for Joann, but she held it together. She carried herself with pride and grace that day. She was the "Mother of the Bride," and you could see she was very happy. She danced with her father and then with each of her brothers.

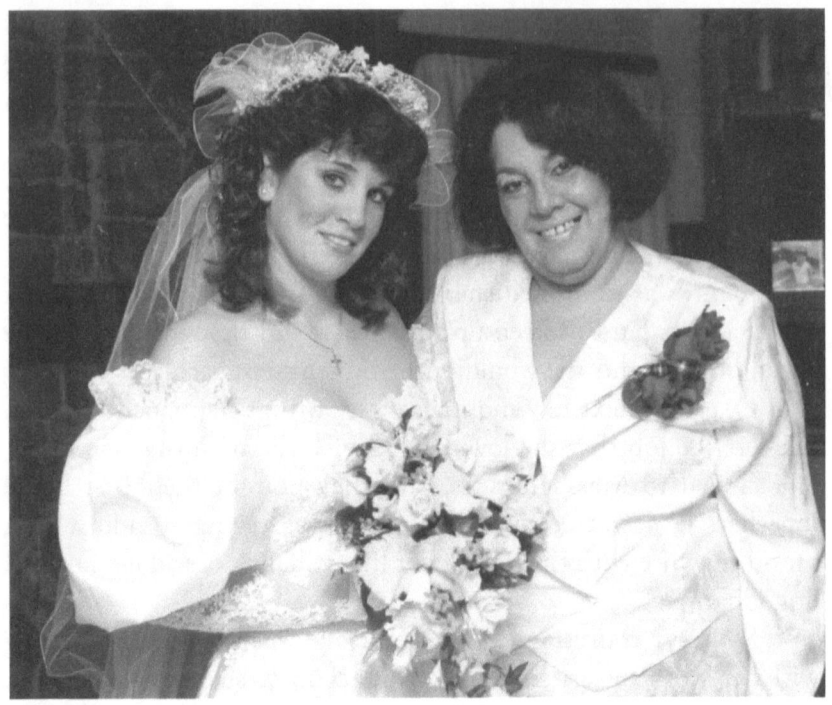

*Lisa›s Wedding November 29, 1986*

Joann felt beautiful in her dress, but why wouldn't she, she wore WHITE!

Joann had to put her mark on the day and insisted on wearing what she called "Winter White." Prior to the wedding, she claimed this color because if her daughter was wearing white so was she. Lisa was not happy about it but let her win the battle. She just wanted a happy day filled with love, and it was.

By the grace of God, Joann held it together as she faced her ex-husband and his new wife and child. She held it together as her only child became a married woman. She even held it together when she had to say goodbye.

Lisa felt like this was a special gift given to her, and that her grandmother was there every step of the way. Lisa felt her throughout the day. When she was standing there talking to her mother, she felt her grandmother touch her wedding dress, the way she said she would. It was a beautiful awestruck moment that Lisa kept to herself; her heart felt full.

Lisa was now a married woman, living in another state. Lisa knew by moving away, that would be the only way she could have some freedom to live. She needed to breathe.

Joann still had her clutches in very deep. You cannot erase the past, or the damage. You can run, but you cannot hide from the darkness. It always finds you.

Joann will never let go, but Lisa now had some ground to stand on.

Distance can give protection to a point.

# Chapter 19

# The Next Stage of Life

Many transitions unfolded over the next few years, and they proved to be quite difficult for Joann and Lisa. The more Joann badgered, displayed poor behaviors, and created drama to gain attention, only put a bigger wedge between mother and daughter. Lisa was quite happy to have an answering machine because when things became too abusive, it was her recording that Joann would lash out on.

The countless messages long, detailed, and extremely vile at times, were what Lisa would come home to after a hard day of work. Even though she could erase it with one flick of the finger, it did not erase the words that had been burned into her mind from the countless years of abuse. The damage festered silently inside her already destroyed heart, brought on by her own mother, the one person who was supposed to love her endlessly. Her own mother could not get past her mental illness that had swallowed her completely.

It was a continued game of cat and mouse as Joann raged on, so angry at her daughter for abandoning her. Joann would remind her daughter of that very thing every chance that she could.

Lisa would always reply the same way, "Mom, I did not abandon you. I moved away. I am always here for you." Lisa remained tough when dealing with her mother, but her insides were crumbling. The many years of dysfunction had taken their toll on her, but she refused to give in to it. Instead, she buried it deep down inside, holding it at bay at all costs.

**Yes, the cost of silence what will that bring?**

Joann and Lisa continued to do this twisted dance of control. The more Joann pushed to gain that control, Lisa would push back just as fierce, becoming more, vile with every episode. At this time in her life, she was now a young mother of three beautiful children. She was trying to keep her home happy and healthy, free of her mother's darkness. She was living her dream of being the mother that she always wanted to have for herself. The balancing act of being a good loving wife, a mother who put her children first always, holding down a job and household proved to be very challenging to say the least. Joann was always in her ear, dropping the guilt card, being extremely demanding, and doing the mental illness dance with the devil.

Finding balance in an extraordinary situation started to break Lisa down. She was pulled in so many different directions and was expected to be first class all the way. There was no room for falter or failure. Lisa worked vigorously to make everyone happy, especially her mother.

Lisa would run down to Connecticut at a moment's notice if her mother truly needed her. When Joann would completely fall apart becoming manic and psychotic, Lisa was right by her side trying to save her from herself. This was a continued journey that they traveled together. It was like a religion. There was no escaping it.

During these turbulent years, Lisa became lost in the madness, continually striving for perfection in all aspects of her life. She was on a mission to prove everyone wrong. She thought by achieving perfection, she could outrun her past. She didn't want to face it! She couldn't face it because the years of abuse beat her into silence. The words would not come out.

So, the old saying, "You can run, but you cannot hide," rang so deeply true.

This was the biggest misconception for Lisa to accept, because the past was on the other end of that phone line every single day since the day she stepped foot out the door of the house up on that hill. A place that held so many memories. The good, the bad, and definitely the ugly.

There were so many times that Lisa would be so enraged by the words of her mother at the other end of that phone line. She would completely absorb every word as it grew larger and larger in front of her face with all sights and sounds becoming distorted. Her heart would race as her face would begin to burn. The distant sound of the children playing in the background sounded like a creepy melody of childhood dreams, and it was at this point Lisa would destroy the telephone ripping it off the wall completely and smashing it to the ground.

SMASH!!!!

It was in those moments that Lisa would be shaken back into reality as her first thoughts went directly back to her children. She hoped and prayed that they did not hear her. By the grace of God, they did not, as they were in the playroom oblivious to the reality their own mother was facing.

As Lisa would hurry to clean up the mess, tears would drip down her face, feeling like she lost control and that could not happen. She was thinking, *How do I once again explain to my husband that another phone has been destroyed due to my own anger?* The anger of a damaged daughter falling victim to the darkness. Many phones were destroyed over the years due to "internal rage."

Finally, the time came when Lisa could not hold it in any longer. The years of abuse, the countless beatings of words by Joann, and the pressures of life brought her to a screeching halt.

Lisa fell apart, and she did it in a very big way. It was time to face her past once and for all. It was time to share with her husband all the dirty details that he did not know. It was time to fill in the pieces of a story that had been "unspoken." John would hear the unspoken truth of the life that Lisa endured many years before they met.

John knew some things, and obviously had to deal with Joann on his own terms, but the darkest part of Lisa's soul would finally come to light. It was a heavy blow for the both of them.

At this point in Lisa's life, she was going to therapy so she could better understand what was happening to her. It was such a frightening experience. She was having anxiety attacks, flashbacks, and nightmares. The nightmares were so brutal that she would wake up screaming and fighting.

Lisa was still living her daily life doing everything she needed to do for her family, but she was living in two worlds at one time. It was a brutal existence. The pain was so heavy, and the anger ran extremely deep. She was muddling through her days, trying to keep it all together. In her mind, all she could think about was freedom and peace.

*How do you escape the darkness?*

Through it all, Joann was still up to her antics creating so much havoc in everyone's lives. It was endless, and nobody could keep up with her. Joann was riding the crazy train, and it was full speed ahead. She could not see the true reality of what was happening, and how her behaviors were affecting her daughter and her family. How could she see the reality with blurred vision?

Lisa took a brief step back during this time to try to regain control of her own life. It was time. With great courage, anxiety, and fear, . . . with the great support of an incredible therapist . . . she was able to share the ugly truth with her husband. It was an atomic bomb to say the least. As the disgusting words rolled from her lips, she would have flashbacks to those awful moments of abuse. Every moment was raw and real as they fell out of her mouth.

John was devastated to hear these words and even said, "Who are you? Do I know you? Did I ever know you?"

It pained Lisa to her very core to hurt the man whom she truly loved with all of her heart and soul, but she had to let the words out to save herself. The burden that she carried for so long was finally flowing from her lips, and once the flood gates opened, it was like a natural disaster.

Husband and wife so in love, being torn apart by these contaminated waters, a cesspool of dirty abuse, and mental illness stewing in a pot of shit! Here it was pouring all over them as they tried to swim to safety, only to be drowning in the muck.

John only knew a part of Lisa. It was the part of her that she took pride in and aspired to be. This was the true Lisa that he fell in love with.

*But who was this other woman, this stranger? Could I ever love* her? Could I ever get beyond feeling betrayed? Will I ever understand her completely, and what else is she hiding from me?*

Oh, the questions, so many questions. Lisa's head was spinning. She knew he had the right to feel the way that he did, but all she could see was anger. Anger that her past brought them here as they spiraled out of control as a couple.

It was a very dark time for both of them as they had to navigate through it all.

Would this make them, or break them? Life still went on! Home life, the children, career, families and of course Joann! It was difficult for both of them, but the one thing that held them together if even only by a thread was love—True Love.

They fought hard as a couple to find their way back to each other, raise a beautiful family and be a strong couple united. They had to fall apart to find one another, and when they did, the pieces began to fall back together. It took many years, many battles and a lot of self-work, but love and commitment won out over hideous abuse.

Lisa also fought hard for her sanity and refused to give in to the silence that almost tore her whole world apart. A world that she wanted more than anything in her entire life. All Lisa ever wanted was a loving husband and a beautiful family. She would not let that go, ever!

Now she had to learn how to navigate the next leg of her journey with her mother. That in itself was a feat that she was not sure she could withstand or overcome.

Time—Time in a bottle—So many stories—So much pain—So many Lessons

Can a mother and daughter ever come together after everything that has happened?

Where do we go from here?

# Chapter 20

# The Cracks

*Note from the Author:*
*There are countless stories that I can share that transpired over the years, but I will share some of the most compelling moments here. My mother and I have been through some unbelievable times in our lives. When I think back to them, it still blows my mind. If I wasn't there experiencing them first hand, I may not have believed it myself. The words that come to mind are profound, outlandish, daunting, and painful.*

*The stories I am about to share are true encounters that happened along the way. Not all moments remembered are good ones; actually many are disturbing, dysfunctional, and sad.*

*It shows how mental illness can cause such damage. This is an illness that cannot always be controlled, and without proper help and support, people fall through the cracks.*

*These stories are the cracks.*

Joann lived life by her rules only! Many of us were railroaded by her laws of life, and the damage runs deep. These stories you are about to read are different moments and personalities of Joann. You never knew who you were going to face!

Growing up with Joann (my mother) proved to be challenging every step of the way. I had to learn at a very young age how to navigate life as I walked this path with her. The one thing that always stood out in my mind, and always will, was how quickly she switched up moods and personalities.

I have spoken and written many times about how I studied her as a young child. I wanted to know where my mom was . . . and if she was going to ever come out of the shell she lived in. I also learned that when her eyes turned black and cold, be afraid!

There were many lessons along the way, that is for sure, but my curiosity to continue to study her lingered on throughout our lives together. I wanted to know who "Joann" really was, and how many personalities lived in one body. Along the way, one thing was quite clear. Joann played hardball. She lived and died by her own rules. She worked hard, played hard, and suffered tremendously as she lived out her life.

I learned that my mom really wanted to be just that, a mom. A loving and caring mother who would die for her children, but mental illness robbed us both of that mother-daughter relationship. It left us with a lifetime of guessing games, abusive situations, and an empty longing for what could never be. I always knew on some level my mother loved me deeply, but her inner demons would never let her come out and play . . . Lisa Zarcone, (Joann's Daughter).

## When You Bring Home A Homeless Man – It Turns Into A Disaster: The Story of Rick

As Joann moved forward with her life, she met many people along the way. Joann was the ultimate vagabond, befriending everyone who was unique, just like her.

At this time in her life, Joann was still driving and living at home with her father. Her mother was now gone, and her daughter was a married woman, who lived out of state.

Joann was a lonely soul and would seek attention wherever and whenever she could claim it. During one of her therapy sessions, she met a man named Rick. He was in the waiting room at DMH (Department of Mental Health), and they started up a conversation. He was a bit younger than her and homeless. This was her type of guy, as she always loved younger men. They bonded instantly and made their way outside to smoke a cigarette, which he of course bummed off of her. Joann lavished in the attention and of course would give the shirt literally off her back, to keep his attention.

Out on the steps in front of DMH is where this dysfunctional relationship blossomed. Of course, he fed her his sob story, and she took the bait hook, line, and sinker. She invited him to come back to her house so she could feed him and care for him. Rick was a shrewd man and played her like a fiddle. He knew he was in!

She brought him home, and her father was less than pleased. They came in loud and boisterous because she was on an instant high, and he followed suit. She explained to her father the situation and stated that Rick could stay with them because he was homeless.

"No Joann he is not staying here. Take him back where you found him," her father said to her.

Joann put up a huge fuss, bullied her father, and shamed him into letting Rick stay the night. Her father angrily agreed.

Joann was in her element. She fed him, had him take a shower, and gave him fresh clothing to wear out of her father's closet. They stayed up all night singing and smoking. Joann never wanted it to end. This was her new man.

The next day, her father lowered the boom. Rick had to go, and a vicious fight emerged. Father and daughter going at it, full throttle.

Joann was not backing down, and Rick sat and watched the show, relishing in the excitement. He was a twisted man who was a true game player. He jumped into the game and started playing on her father's heartstrings, until he once again was brow beaten down to allowing the madness to continue.

Joann took her father's money to buy more cigarettes and beer for her new friend. They also bought a bunch of food and just partied on for three days, until her father could not take it another minute longer. He called in the troops!

He called his daughter and son. He asked them to come up to the house and help him get rid of this awful man. Then he called his granddaughter Lisa, explained the situation, and asked for her help as well.

"If she will listen to anyone Lisa, it would be you. Please come down for a visit. I need your help," her grandfather begged.

With disgust and contempt in her voice, Lisa stated, "I will be down tomorrow."

This was not the first time Lisa would have to drop everything in her life to drive to Connecticut so she could deal with her mother's antics. Unfortunately, this was a pattern that carried out repeatedly though-out her adult life with Joann.

The dysfunction raged on . . .

As the partying continued, Joann went head-to-head with her brother and sister, spewing her vile words of hate onto both of them. She even became physical with her brother and his wife. She picked up her sister-in-law and threw her. She pushed her brother out the back door, as Rick watched in delight. Her sister came in for round two.

Joann was ready for her, and they went at it verbally! Her father felt like a prisoner in his own home and was not mentally strong enough to battle Joann alone. Her sister gave her an ultimatum. "Get him out of here by the end of the day or you are out as well! This is daddy's house, not yours!"

Joann went out of her mind screaming and throwing things so ferociously, with pure violence and hate, that her sister turned around and walked out.

The next day proved to be a bit different when her daughter arrived. Joann was cool as a cucumber, but her eyes and sarcasm showed another side of her.

In two days, Joann displayed many personalities—Mania—Sex Kitten—Violence—Distraught Victim—and devastated mother.

Lisa knew instantly as she walked through the door that her mom was ready to battle. Joann was completely manic, talking so fast you could not understand a word that she was saying. She was spitting, swearing, and then crying.

Lisa just stood there and let her have her moment, then she directed her attention to her grandfather giving him a hug and kiss. She held his hands and said, "I will handle this."

"Ohhh YEAHHHH! Lisa handles everything!" Joann snorted with her voice husky and heavy. "I am your mother, and what I say goes. You hear me you snotty little bitch!"

Lisa completely ignored her mother's vile words and turned her attention to the man sitting in the chair with a smirk on his face.

"You must be Rick," Lisa said.

"Oh yes I am," he said with a coy smile.

"OK Rick, here it is. I will be blunt! You need to leave today, as you have overstayed your welcome. You have no right to be in a place where you do not belong, taking advantage of my mother and grandfather. If you do not leave, I will call the police and have your ass dragged out of here. So do us all a favor and get out."

As the last words flowed from Lisa's lips, her mom went on the attack!

"Who the fuck do you think you are coming in here talking to him like that! Get the fuck out of here!" Joann was screaming so fiercely she wet her pants. As the urine continued to poor down her legs, she continued to yell.

Lisa stood there with a look of—*You are not going to win this battle—Not this time!*

"Enough is enough, he is out whether you like it or not," Lisa said and looked at Rick. "What are you going to do? Make a choice."

He got up and grabbed a hold of Joann and said, "It is time for me to go. Your family doesn't want me here. I will be in the car." He grabbed his stuff and walked out.

Joann turned all of her anger onto her daughter, shoving her across the room.

Lisa's grandfather got in between them, and Joann screamed at her, "You are dead to me! You hear me, dead!" She grabbed her pocketbook and keys, and stormed out the door.

As she was racing to the car, Lisa stuck her head out the door and screamed at her, "I will be waiting for you, when you come back."

Joann gave her the finger, jumped in the car, and backed out of the driveway like a madwoman.

Lisa and her grandfather listened to her peel out all the way down the street, and then they sat at the famous kitchen table and waited for her to return. They both knew she would come back because she couldn't wait for another round of arguments with her daughter.

As they sat there and talked, Lisa prepared herself for the next battle.

"Thank you, Lisa, for coming. I knew she would listen to you," her grandfather said with a voice of exhaustion.

"We will see how long it lasts, grandpa, but I know she will come back alone."

It was about four hours later when Joann finally returned home, smelling of dried-up urine and cigarettes. Her mascara was running down her face, and they couldn't tell of it was from crying or something else.

As they sat and had a long-drawn-out conversation, Joann never shared what happened during those four hours, but whatever it was, they could tell it was completely wild and out of control.

Time moved forward, and Joann continued to bring Rick around and he warmed up to her father. Joann's dad gave up fighting with her and allowed Rick to come and go as he pleased. Eventually, Rick (who was homeless), pitched his tent in the field far back on the property. For a while it worked out, as nobody knew he was there.

Joann enjoyed spending time with this strange man and bestowed him with an abundance of attention. The scenarios and antics became too much for her father to handle. Many disturbing things were beginning to happen, and his home felt out of control. He became increasingly distraught by the situation and broke down. Once again, he called in the troops!

One by one family members came, and Joann fought a vicious battle with each and every one of them. She would not back down, as the battles raged on. At times it became violent, and Rick was enjoying the entertainment.

Lisa once again made the trip down to her grandfather's home to try and help out. This time she came with her husband. When they got there, Joann was nowhere to be found. Lisa and John sat with her grandfather, and he updated them on the situation.

When Joann finally returned home, she was manic and hysterical.

"Rick raped me! Rick raped me!" she was screaming.

Lisa went into panic mode. Just that word alone was a huge trigger for her because of her damaging past. Lisa started screaming, "Oh my God, what are you saying mom?"

"Rick raped me in the tent, that is where I was. I told him to stop and he didn't."

As Joann sobbed uncontrollably, Lisa spotted Rick coming down the hill, and she went running. Her husband and grandfather followed behind her. She ran up to him screaming in his face, "Did you rape my mother you mother fucker!"

He looked Lisa straight in the eye and said, "No I did not, she wanted it!"

"Get the fuck out of her now you piece of shit and never come back because I am calling the police!"

Rick starting spewing a bunch of bullshit and made his way down the driveway in a panic.

They all turned around quickly, rushing back into the house, as they wanted to make sense out of this complete mess. Nobody knew what to really think, but they needed answers. Lisa began to ask her mother questions, and she repeated it all.

"Rick raped me."

"I am calling the police, and we will have him arrested."

When the police arrived, Joann changed her tune. She became combative and aggressive toward the police officers. This had now turned into another shit show, in itself. Joann was so out of control, that her behaviors got her a one-way trip to the hospital.

Here came Joann, back to the psychiatric unit. When she got there, she tore up the place. She went completely ballistic! Sadly, she was restrained and drugged to calm her down. Oh, the pattern! This display was a repeat cycle of dysfunction. Joann was the revolving door patient, and they all knew her name.

Lisa showed up a little while later. As she walked those halls with her husband by her side, she could feel that sick pit in her stomach. The one that she always felt every time, when Joann was locked up!

Lisa was silently thinking, *How many times must we do this dance, and how much more can I bear without breaking?*

Her husband squeezed her hand as they walked through the locked doors. Once inside Lisa felt like she could not breathe; everything was tight inside of her.

The nurse gave her the lowdown of what had transpired, and as she spoke, the words became muffled and drowned out.

Hit that repeat button, blah blah blah, This is what Lisa was feeling right in that moment because it was so repetitive. After their conversation, they went in to check on her mom. There she was tied to the bed, beaten, bruised, and whimpering.

Lisa approached her, "Mom it is me. I am here."

She started sobbing, "Lisa, Lisa, Lisa, help me! Oh my God, please help me!"

"Mom, rest for now and we will work on getting you out of here soon. Please just rest now."

As Joann continued to sob, John stood in the corner, watching with this uncomfortable and distraught look on his face. He hated to see her mom like this, and it broke his heart that there was nothing he could do to help his wife, except for just be there. It tore him up every single time. John loved Lisa so deeply, and he chose to ride that crazy rollercoaster with her. He wanted to protect her any way that he could.

Lisa looked back at him with tears in her eyes, and he gave her a wink. Lisa turned back to her mom and said, "I love you mom. It will be ok."

Joann fell asleep. Lisa left instructions at the front desk, and they left to go back to her grandfather's.

As they walked out hand in hand, Lisa appreciated the support of her husband. For years nobody was there for her, truly there for her, but he was in every sense of the word. Walking down that hall, hearing the sounds of their own footsteps, Lisa made a detour for the chapel. They both went inside and sat. Lisa prayed so deeply for her mother, and so did John.

Once they made their way out of the hospital, Lisa turned to him and said, "At least I know she is safe for now. Thank you for coming with me. I love you."

"I love you too," John responded.

After all the dysfunction and madness, Joann retracted her statement about the rape. She spent four weeks in the hospital, and upon returning home, rekindled her friendship with Rick. He was no longer welcome at the house, but she would go visit him and his new girlfriend, Valerie.

Sometimes, Joann would spend days there, and nobody knew what truly was going on but Joann herself. She never shared the dirty details, and honestly Lisa didn't want to know. Lisa just wanted her mother safe.

This friendship between Joann and Rick lasted for years. He eventually moved out of state with his girlfriend, but he called Joann regularly until he passed away.

Was Joann raped on that fateful day or was it sex in a tent?
We never found out the true story.

This Union:
Connected by illness, bound by dysfunction, loyal to the end!

**Joann Moves Out—**

After the passing of her father, Joann stayed on at the family home on the hill, until it was time to eventually move forward.

The ground work that went into finding the right place for Joann was daunting and long winded. Lisa advocated for her mother every step of the way, making sure she would be able to live comfortably and have the proper help and support that she would need to be on her own.

Throughout Joann's whole life, she had never lived alone. Finally, after all these years, she would get her chance. What would she do with her new found freedom? With no family members looking over her shoulder!

Joann spent the next ten years of her life making countless mistakes, taking far too many risks, and creating havoc every step of the way. She tortured her daughter with the things that she was doing out there on her own. Joann was wild to the core, and stepped into the path of freedom with total fury. She was at the highest of the highs and the lowest of the lows.

Lisa received countless phone calls over the years in regards to her mother's behaviors, and drove endless miles back and forth between Massachusetts and Connecticut, trying to save Joann from herself. It was mentally and emotionally exhausting for Lisa to keep up with her mother's antics, but she stayed vigilant as she marched by her side every step of the way, always her true advocate.

**Joann's Time Living By The Ocean . . . An Ocean View**

Joann loved the ocean, the smells and the sounds that came from the beach walk. There was always action and entertainment, which was right up her alley. She moved into a highrise on the water for the over fifty crowd, who needed assistance. She lived on the seventh floor in Apartment 130. It was a cute little apartment, and the view from her window gave her comfort as the church was right next door. To the right was the beach walk with the ocean in the backdrop.

The church bells rang daily and played beautiful music, which she enjoyed. The religious side of Joann (this personality) was very deep in her faith. She would cry and pray daily. She would speak to Jesus and call him her friend. In times of distress, she would curse him for bringing her such pain but vowed to always walk besides him.

Then there was the other side of Joann. The woman who just wanted to have endless fun. When the music from the beach walk would makes its way through her window, as the salty sea air followed, she would switch gears. Joann would make her way downstairs and out those doors. She had an electric wheelchair, so she would put it in high gear making her way down to the water. She was fueled by the energy of the crowds, loud music, and endless action. You could say she was in her element.

Joann would smoke, mingle with the people, and sing loudly! She made many friends down by the water and in her apartment building. You could say Joann was a celebrity down there, and everyone knew her name.

Of course, along the way, Joann made sure she was connecting with the men. She loved attention and made sure she was getting it. She did make friends with some of the women who lived in her apartment building, but she made many enemies as well.

When Joann's "Sex Kitten" side came out (she liked to refer to herself as that or a "Vixen"), her sensual nature came shining on through, and many of the older women didn't like the way she would talk to their husbands.

Joann would teeter on being completely vulgar at times. Of course the horny old men loved it, but to the wives, she was called a whore, or in "old terms" a Jezebel. When Lisa would come down to visit her mother with the children, she would always get an earful from the tenants by the sea.

Oh, Joann could be a bad bad girl!

Lisa would be sickened by the tales that were being told and tried to keep her mother in check, but how could she? She lived far away, but the phone calls from the property manager were constant, as well as from the mental health staff and nurses. It was a constant battle of the wills, and the calls would come in day and night. Lisa was always trying to bridge the gap between the many moods and outrageous behaviors of her mother.

Things would always become worse when Joann would take

herself off of her medications. She was either miraculously cured of all mental illness, or she was allergic to the medicines. There were many reasons why she would do it, but the saddest reason of all was when she would say, "I just want to feel, these medicines make me numb, and I feel no love in my heart." Those words were heartbreaking to hear, but at the same time there could never be balance. It was either one way or the other. This is what mental illness does to so many people! It is a never-ending journey of trying to keep balance and maintain control of thoughts, emotions, and actions. You have to put in the work every single day, and that becomes exhausting. For Joann it felt like entrapment.

Joann wanted to be Joann, and every day that was someone different.

The sobbing phone calls to her daughter would become out of control, with phone calls exceeding ten times in one day. Lisa always knew when the downward spiral was upon them. It always started out the same way.

First it would be the great depression. The crying, out of control sobbing, and the deep heavy feelings of death. During these times, Joann would lay in her bed for days, smoking her cigarettes, urinating all over herself, and refusing to shower. Due to her incontinence issues, she was supposed to wear "her diaper" as she called it, but would refuse. She hated wearing them, and who could blame her, but the alternatives it was sitting in urine! She would develop the worst rashes on her skin. It was also dangerous for her because she was a diabetic, who did not take care of herself properly. That was a whole other battle that went on for years.

After she would emotionally beat herself up, and everyone she came in contact with, the tides would change.

Second it would be Manic Mode!

Joann would go from a deep depression to an ultimate high. Her mood would change completely. Her demeanor would shift, along with her clothing. She would go into "over sexual" mode, and this was the dangerous side of her.

She had a wardrobe for all of her different moods.

Once in Manic Mode off came the bra and conservative clothing, and on came the tube tops and elastic waisted bohemian skirts with NO underwear.

Joann would lay in the grass on the front lawn of her apartment complex, and in the worst of times, hike up her skirt when not wearing any underwear. She would scream obscenities as people passed on by. It was a disturbing display, which either resulted in the police coming to get her, or her daughter.

Lisa confronted her mother in those disturbing moments many times, encouraging her to get up off the ground on her own terms so she wouldn't be arrested. In those moments, Joann loved the battle and made it very difficult for everyone, especially her daughter. It was mentally exhausting trying to keep up with her!

*Run Lisa Run*, were her mother's words always playing in her mind. "Oh Lisa so uptight, you can never take a joke!"

The mindset of Joann during her manic times!

## Going to The Chapel—
## A Complex Relationship Between Mother and Daughter

It was a hot summer day, and I was busy running with the children. It was summer vacation, and our lives were filled with high energy. They say during the summer time schedules get lighter, but not when you have a house filled with children and their friends! My husband and I created a happy safe home filled with chaos and laughter. We were the safe house for all the children in the neighborhood who were not as lucky as our crew. My past had taught me that not all homes are safe and comfortable like ours.

As the phone rings, I pick it up, and the voice on the other end brings me right back to that time in my life when all was dark!

Before I could finish the word hello, my mother was frantically screaming at me so loud that I had to pull the phone away from my ear so I did not become instantly deaf! Her fast-paced manic tone told me instantly that my mother was off in a very bad way, and me her devoted daughter, was going to go on another countless emotional ride to hell. As I tried to calm her down and understand what was happening, I heard her screaming and then another voice came on the phone.

"Hello, is this Lisa Zarcone?" the man asks.

Of course I say, "Yes."

"I am a police officer, and we have come to take your mother to the hospital, as there have been many complaints about her out of control behavior.

My heart instantly sinks, as I know all too well what that means. I continue to hear her screaming bloody murder in the background. My eyes well up, and instantly I am thrust into a flashback of a moment in time when I was a young girl watching the police drag her away kicking, screaming, and fighting for her life. This disturbing image is haunting!

I compose myself and ask that they take her to St. Raphael's Hospital in New Haven, Connecticut, as they know her there, and she will get the help that she needs. You see my mother was what they call the "revolving door" patient in Celentano 1 (the psychiatric unit). My mother was severely mentally ill and struggled for years with this disease. There were times in her life when she would take herself off her medication, and the downward spiral would begin.

Here we are again! I ask the police officer on the phone to please try to be kind to her as she is a very sick woman. He told me they would try, but unfortunately when my mother was in this state on mind, she was violent. I have been on the other end of the violence too many times to mention, and every nerve inside my body was now shaking as I fight off the flashbacks of the past to stay in control of my own emotions.

My house was filled with innocent children, and they do not need to be connected to that in any way . . . the forever balancing act of an abuse survivor. I was living in two worlds at the same time, trying to do it all, and keep my own personal feelings and thoughts under wraps.

This takes a toll on the brain after years of being beaten down by old patterns that die hard. The words placed upon me by my own mother drip from my soul, tainting me with scars so thick you could never see through it toward the light of day.

MY SILENCE . . . UNSPOKEN . . .

I contact my husband and ask for him to come home and take over so that I can make my way down to Connecticut and handle the situation. I needed to make sure that my mother was ok. You see I was her forever advocate, as so many others left her to the wayside, and I was left holding the bag!

My ride down from Massachusetts to Connecticut was always

the same during these trying times. My mind would wander to the past, with old memories flooding back to taunt me. I tried to focus while I drove, but it was nearly impossible.

Oh my God . . . this pattern that I relive repeatedly each time she ends up back in the hospital was always the same. I am angry, distraught, worried for her safety, and guilty on every level because I should be able to save my mother, right? This is what my past has done to me!

As I made my way through the hospital, I knew the exact path to take, walking those steps, hearing the loud stomping of my own feet as my heart raced out of control, pounding in my ears. I briefly looked over at the big paintings on the wall of the priests, nuns, and doctors of the past. Their eyes are staring at me glaring like to say, "YOU AGAIN!" and in my head I say back "YES ME!"

The door to the chapel is glowing, illuminating with light shining on in the middle of this insane darkness. I whisper, "I will be back soon."

I hit the buzzer, announce who I am and ask if I can come in to talk about my mother Joann.

The nurse of the other end says, "Ok Lisa come in." She knows me by my first name! Now, that says it all right there. I made my way to the nurse's station where we have a brief chat about what's happened and then she takes me to my mother.

There she is, my mother sitting in a chair talking to herself, as she is crying, swearing, and spitting on the ground, spewing such vulgarity that you would never think such a devout catholic woman would ever say out loud!

As I stand there just taking it all in, she turns her head with this evil glare in her eyes and says to me, "Are you here to take me home, you bitch?"

I calmly say, "No mom, not today."

Then she unleashed her vile banter onto me with such force, my insides shake to the core of my soul. When she was done screaming so loud that she peed her pants, as well as the floor, she sat in her urine and started to sing this crazy song about a monkey's asshole, waving her arms in the air instantly high as a kite; fueled by the manic energy bursting at every seam. I stand there in horror. I have witnessed this display many times before, and it never lessens the pain in the moment, it enhances it each time I see it. My insides scream as my inner child weeps for protection, but my outer shell is tough as nails as I manage to get out the words that need to be said in that moment.

When it is time to go, it's back to vulgarity, blame, hateful words, and tears. She weeps, screaming at God, "Why do you have to be so cruel? I am your best friend. Why do you continue to hurt me!" Screaming, even louder, for her only son now in the hands of the lord. It's a very sad and disturbing display to witness when all you want is your mother to be OK. All you want is your mother to be your mother, but in reality, I am the mother! I am the caregiver, protector, diligent daughter/mother all in one. I kiss her on the forehead as she weeps, and I leave.

I make sure that the doctors and nurses are all on the same page, and that they have all my information to contact me. I assured them that I will be calling in later, and I will definitely be back. I always made sure that my mother was cared for the best way possible. It was hard being her daughter.

As I walked out the door and heard it slam and lock behind me, tears well up in my eyes, that old familiar pain seeps out of me. As I walk, I make my way to that chapel door and sit up front closest to the alter. There is nobody in there, and I am grateful. I feel the angels always knew when I needed alone time with God. I weep silently and share my most inner thoughts with this intense spirit that I feel moving through me. I always ask why, and what do I need to do next? I drop to my knees and pray.

I pray for strength, courage, and the inner faith to see us both through another battle that continually tears us apart. Mother and daughter are connected by a love line never to be broken, that is being chipped away by an illness that is bigger than both of us. I ask for forgiveness for anything I may have done wrong in my life to deserve this, then I sit in silence and wait. I wait for answers. I wait for calmness and peace.

As I close my eyes, I feel wind blowing over me, cool and calming. I breathe it in as the tears begin to flow harder, and more intense. Then it all stops.

As the lights flicker in this little chapel of peace, I am OK. I get up and make my way to the door holding on to my faith with all my might. As I make my way down the hall, I look at those paintings and I say, "Watch over my mom. I love her, and she needs to be ok." Then I leave, making my way back home to my family who needs me.

I am torn between two worlds every day of my life, and my faith is what has seen me through it all. I am the constant juggler.

# Chapter 21

# Off To The Nursing Home— The Next Stage Of Life

After countless trials and tribulations over the years, which included a kitchen fire, a mattress fire, and Joann burning her stomach three times with hot boiling water, the state deemed her incompetent to live home alone even though she had assistance.

She hit the point of no return and could not be trusted or safe in her own surroundings. This was a hard pill for Joann to swallow, as she loved her freedom and her apartment by the ocean. This was her spot, and she put up a gallant fight to the bitter end before she accepted the fact that it was time to move forward.

Finding Joann a nursing home that fit her needs was quite difficult for many reasons, but the top issue was her smoking. Joann smoked all day and night, and living in a nursing home would interrupt her insatiable need to have her cigarettes close at hand.

Joann lived in three different nursing homes before finding her final destination in Hamden, Conneticut. We did find her a spot that had an open courtyard, which offered her many of the things that she enjoyed. She could go out there freely, enjoy the company of others, and have her diet soda as she smoked away. She called that her peaceful times. She loved to bring out bread and crackers to feed the birds and enjoyed the beautiful flowers.

Even though she missed her apartment and the ocean deeply, she made the best of her surroundings. Joann talked like she was a politician at times, stating "My People need me, and I am the voice for the elderly!" She felt like she was the voice for everyone and would become argumentative at the drop of a dime if she felt the need to defend herself or anyone else that she felt was being wronged.

This behavior did get her into a lot of hot water, and her daughter received quite a few phone calls in regards to her combative behaviors. Joann even had a fist fight with her roommate, a ninety-three-year-old woman who would always give her a difficult time. One night it all came to a head, and the roommate put her hands on Joann. She was not having it and a brawl began. Joann was not afraid to fight that was for sure, and her past had taught her to protect herself at all costs.

The end result, Joann got her own room and was quite happy about this arrangement. She could decorate it as she pleased and created a whole little world that only made sense to her! The only other person that could figure out the rhyme and reason to this disastrous mess was her daughter. As Lisa would sit on the floor cutting big pieces of colorful yarn stuck in the wheels of Joann's wheel chair, she would look around at the madness. She understood it because this was her life growing up. This is what she was exposed to for countless years!

The creative yarn dolls, tinfoil, ribbons, and pictures taped on the wall told a very telling tale of Joann's life and her mental status. She lived in the past, in a clouded world of sadness and sorrow. When she was angry, she would rip pictures into shreds, then tape them back together. She cut people out of certain photos because of the wrongs they had done to her along the way. She lived like a gypsy, and that was how she felt! She dressed in a very unique way, and one would think she was homeless because of her style.

Her daughter would become quite frustrated with her because she always gave her things away. All of her new clothing, hats, jackets—everything gone! Lisa would come down to visit and see other residents go by with her mother's belongings on. Lisa knew it was her mother's items because she labeled everything, trying to curb the freebies Joann offered out into the world.

When Lisa would question her mother, she was met with

sarcasm and nasty comments. Then Joann would go on to tell people that "her daughter" never brings her anything! Oh, the battles, they were ongoing and endless!

Lisa could not keep up with her mom's insatiable need to give EVERYTHING away. It became even harder when Joann was not stable, because she would accuse people of stealing. She would start many arguments with staff and other residents during these times of struggle.

Even though Joann was in a nursing home, she still rode the mental health rollercoaster and would refuse her meds quite frequently. They could not force her to take her medications, so Joann ran the show! There was always a struggle, a battle, many harsh words, and countless tears.

Overall, the staff was very good to her even when she was at her worst. They would go out of their way to help her, and at times when Joann was paranoid and untrusting, her vicious side would come out. She sent many staff out of her room crying because of how difficult she would become.

Joann was a die-hard. It didn't matter how educated or seasoned a doctor, nurse, or staff member was, Joann knew how to go for the jugular and would do so in moment's notice. Lisa had been on the other end of that nastiness pretty much her whole life, so when she would receive the phone calls pertaining to her mother's "awful behaviors," nothing surprised her. She would explain how she could be, offer the best advice that she could, and in the end, Joann was doing what she wanted to do.

She always said she had zero freedom and no control, but the reality was, she knew exactly what she was doing, maintained control and put everyone else in their place, including her daughter. It was her world, and nobody was going to make the calls except for her. When she didn't get her way, watch out. It was a complete explosion and the ultimate battle of the wills.

When Joann lost a battle, you could bet your life everyone would pay the price, especially her daughter. Being the daughter of Joann was not for the faint of heart, and Lisa had to be tough as nails, wear a hard-core shell, and battle through it like a warrior. There was no time for tears, weakness, or rest. It was an ongoing battle every single day in the life path of Joann and Lisa.

As time moved forward, there were also many trips to the hospital when Joann would hit a complete low and bottom out. There was a psychiatric hospital close by that dealt with geriatric patients. This was Joann's new revolving door unit that she would be placed in when it all became too much.

Lisa shifted gears in her thoughts, actions, and behaviors when it came to her mother, as she was learning how to understand her a bit better. Lisa was also seeking therapy to weed through her own damage, trauma, and pain. It was there that she found understanding for her mother's illness. It was also in therapy where Lisa learned how to separate her mother from the illness. It was a long painstaking process that opened countless dark doors of the past. As Lisa learned to heal from within, she was learning to love her mother on a deeper level.

This process took years to achieve, and with that being said, there were still many moments that brought her right back to her childhood. The old pings of the past could still sting like a bee every time. Trying to find balance with all of these thoughts and emotions proved to be difficult for a long time to come. The hardest part was going to visit her mom in the hospital. When Joann was at her extreme worst, it would break Lisa's heart every single time. It also triggered everything in her body as her anxiety would rise as she traveled up the elevator to the fourth floor. It was there that all of her inner work would fall to crap.

Like a thief in the night, it would claim her of all balance and grounding. It was a free for all of shame, blame, anger, and sadness. A lethal bomb ready to blow, as she tried with every ounce of her being to hold it all together.

Her outer shell was tight, but her insides were exploding!

There was one particular visit that affected Lisa and her husband greatly. There was many things happening with Joann at this time in her life which brought her to an even darker place, if you can imagine that.

**Here is the imagery . . .**

As John and Lisa take the hour-long trek down to the hospital, they were in deep conversation about what the future may hold for Joann. This was always a difficult conversation, which left Lisa feeling angry and upset. John was a very realistic person who always helped Lisa put things into perspective, but not without controversy between husband and wife.

Joann always had a magical way of putting a monkey wrench into their relationship. Their marriage and life together had an extra stress, which put a deep strain on their relationship, and that extra stress was Joann. Lisa had deep loyalty to her husband and children, but she also had a profound loyalty and never-ending duty to her mother. In spite of all that happened in life, Lisa remained loyal every step of the way.

John struggled with this for many years, but over time became more understanding of her circumstances. This particular visit gave him a whole new understanding, compassion, and sadness for his mother-in-law, whom he truly loved as well.

As they made their way into the building and up that elevator, there was an eerie silence between them. Lisa was internally shaking as her anxiety was rising. She was thinking of the last words the doctor told her on the phone, "Your mother has hit another level of her mental illness, and we feel she has some dementia settling in the mix of her mania."

*How much more can she take? How much more could her mother's mind and body tolerate?* Lisa thought. This was a mixed bag of emotions to swallow.

As they made their way to the door, Lisa hit the buzzer to be let in. The nurse Shirley greets them with a smile and a somber look at the same time. They stand in the hallway and chat before visiting Joann. Shirley went on to say it had been a really bad morning, and Joann was now sitting in the atrium staring at the wall.

Stepping forward onto the unit was very hard. As John and Lisa walked by each doorway, there was a patient either in bed moaning and screaming or sitting in a wheel chair at the doorway hunched over drooling. It was a very sad sight indeed. As they made their way further, they could smell shit, YES, shit. The stench was overwhelming and made you want to instantly gag.

They were stopped briefly in the hallway as nurses and doctors went charging into a room to handle a patient who decided to paint the walls with his own poop, as he was eating it. This was sad and disturbing to witness.

Once we were allowed to finally pass through the third set of locked doors, we made it into the atrium. This was a big bright beautiful room with high ceilings, sky lights, and a picture-perfect view of the mountains out the extra-large picture window.

There was a lot of activity all around. Some residents were watching tv, others were at the big community table doing arts and crafts. There was even a patio area outside where people could go sit among all the beautiful flowers. The energy was high, active, and engaging—but not for Joann. The nurse pointed to the corner of the room.

Lisa was holding John's hand and squeezed it so tight. The overwhelming amount of sadness that washed over her was unbearable.

As they made their way closer, they could hear her speaking. Who was Joann talking to?

Lisa and John just stood close for a moment to really listen, and what they heard was heartbreaking to say the least. Joann was talking to Jesus. In one breath she was telling him how much she loved him, and asked, "Why do you continue to let me suffer. I am your friend." Then in the next breath, she was angry as she raised her fists in the air cursing him for taking her only son and she wished the devil upon him.

This was a cycle she just repeated over and over.

Lisa found the courage from within to step forward so her mom could see her.

With a half-smile, Lisa said, "Mom, hi it is me. I am here. What is going on?"

Joann looked up at her, and in that moment, she looked like a lost child painfully broken, and Lisa's heart sank. As her mother stared at her for a bit, her face changed. It was horrifying as her eyes went from sadness to extreme anger.

Lisa took a step back as Joann started to swat at her, cursing such vulgarity. She then shifted her eyes to John and called him a "Mother Fucking Prick who took her daughter away from her." She compared him to Jesus who stole her son. As they stood there listening to the badgering, Lisa stepped forward once again and grabbed her mother's hand.

"Mom, Mom. Stop it, we are here! Do you see us? We are here for you, please stop it!"

Switching gears quickly, Joann responded snidely, "Oh poor Mona Lisa you could never take a joke." As she looked beyond her daughter, she said to John, "Let's go outside and have a smoke."

John replied, "Not today, Joann, not today."

Joann turned back to the wall and engaged in the same conversation she was having when they got there and completely ignored them. The nurse came over to try to help the situation, but it only made it worse. Joann was now crying uncontrollably as she prayed out loud. She just repeated this process over and over again.

Lisa and John stayed for a very long time that day, trying to get her to engage, but it was an epic failure. When they left, Lisa felt defeated and distraught. John tried to comfort her the best way that he knew how, but the past damage had put Lisa in to a headspace that was very unhealthy.

When visits like this happened, it took Lisa a very long time to overcome them, as the internal movie theater in her mind would repeat the stories from the past, and that pain ate away at her.

Post Traumatic Stress Disorder (PTSD) at its finest.

Again, putting strain on her marriage, Lisa went back to therapy, as she knew she needed help with this heavy load. Trying to live a full life with one foot in the past had become too much for her to bear.

Time to weed through the rubble!

This was again another painful process to endure as she still had the duties of wife, mother, and advocate for her mom. The pressure and stress were astounding, and at times she felt like she would completely fall apart. In her mind she needed peace and freedom from all of it. The balancing act was a hard role to play.

Joann was not bouncing back as quickly as she normally would, so Lisa received a very difficult phone call from the hospital. They wanted Lisa to become conservator for her mother. This is something that Lisa truly did not want to do because of the repercussions and added guilt from her mother.

The hospital told her if she did not want to do it, then they would request to have one set in place for her. Lisa knew that was not the answer, and she did not trust strangers with the fate of her mom. She knew all too well how mentally ill people fall through the cracks, and the treatment that could be bestowed upon them because of foul behaviors.

Once again Lisa stepped up, and said she would do it. After all the preparatory work was complete, Lisa had to go down to the hospital for a hearing. An attorney was assigned to her, but there was also an attorney assigned to Joann.

Joann was livid with her daughter for agreeing to the conservatorship, and even after Lisa tried repeatedly to explain to her why she stepped forward, in Joann's eyes it was a complete betrayal. Joann let her daughter have it right to the core and didn't hold back, destroying Lisa with her vicious words. Lisa took it as she sat in silence and allowed her mother to just let it out. She was dying on the inside as internal rage echoed in her ears, but as she stared at her mother, nobody had a clue of the "inner reality."

The judge then came in and asked Lisa questions, and then Joann. The lawyer for Joann stepped forward next and barreled Lisa with awful accusations and unnecessary questioning, as he tried to make Lisa out to be the villain in all of this. He was there for Joann that was for sure, and he went toe to toe with Lisa. It got to such a vile point, that the judge finally put an end to the questioning, asking the lawyer what he thought he was gaining by tearing Joann's daughter apart!

The lawyer's response was, "I am just representing my client to the fullest extent, as she asked of me."

Lisa was sitting there like a statue, no movement, no sign of emotion. All the prep work from her past came flooding forward to guide her through another horrifying situation.

When it was over and the judge granted conservatorship to Lisa, Joann stood up and cursed her daughter screaming, "Die bitch, Die! You are dead to me now!" as the nurses dragged her away.

Lisa then stood up and looked the lawyer in the eyes and said, "Do you think you're a big man now? I bet you're feeling really good about yourself! You are a complete asshole!"

He responded with, "I was doing my job, no hard feelings."

Before Lisa could respond back, her lawyer said to him, "How dare you treat my client in such a way. I will be filing a complaint due to your abusive actions."

Joann's lawyer just chuckled and walked away.

At that moment, Lisa fell back into the chair shaking uncontrollably. The tears began to flow, and she had never felt so alone in her life. Everyone was staring at her, but nobody offered any condolences or comfort, except Shirley, the nurse who walked over, took Lisa by the hand, and escorted her into the other room. She gave Lisa her time to grieve and pull herself back together.

After a period of time, Lisa emerged and found Shirley. She thanked her for her kindness, and they had a heartfelt conversation. Lisa then went back in to see her mother one more time before leaving.

Again, Lisa tried to explain to Joann about why she stepped in, but Joann didn't want to hear it.

"Mom it would be better for you if they go through me, not a stranger. I know you better than anyone. I love you and have your best interest at heart always."

Joann looked her in the eye and said, "Get out! I hate you! I will see you in hell."

"Well take a good look because that is where we are right now. Mom, they will send you back to the nursing home, and you can be with your people. You can smoke, drink your soda and coffee, and enjoy the things you love. This step forward is getting you out of here."

"Yaa Yaa," is all Joann replied and dismissed her daughter once again.

Lisa got up and walked toward the door, giving one last glance before leaving. Joann completely ignored her.

Lisa quietly inside her mind said, *God please protect my mom and allow her to forgive me. I love her and just want her safe.*

Lisa let out a deep sigh and walked out of the room. She saw Shirley once again, and they exchanged a few words, then she left. The drive home that day was a mixed bag of emotions with intense sorrow and guilt. Lisa knew she did the right thing, but as always, it came with a price tag.

Once everything settled down, Joann returned to the nursing home and back to her private room. She was surrounded by all of her favorite things, and even if she never admitted to it, Lisa knew she was happy. That was her sanctuary among the rubble of HER past. The old clothing, the pictures hanging on the wall, the old Samsonite hard turquoise suitcase that she stored her yarn in, and the statues her angels.

She was home.

# Chapter 22

# The Damaged Relationship

Time in a Bottle . . . the past floated along endlessly, crashing into the present over and over again until the glass was completely broken. This is how Lisa felt about her relationship with her mother.

All she ever wanted in life was her mom to "be a mom," and what she got was a raw deal with a lifetime of hurt and pain.

*How do you find love in that pile of disaster?*

That was the biggest question Lisa had to ask herself, and it was the hardest one to weed through. In therapy Lisa truly did the work . . . as devastating as it was . . . she did it. She pushed through all the painful memories of the past, so again she could find her mother and their connection.

**The Next Leg Of Her Journey**

Joann settled back into her surroundings and was back to calling her daughter for a visit. Lisa made her way down to Connecticut as often as possible, bringing her mother all that she asked for and needed. The more Lisa worked on herself, she once again saw her mother in a clearer light. It was hard work to separate the illness from her mother, but it was there that she got glimpses of love from her mother. It was also there that Lisa realized she had a lot of great qualities that Joann had.

Strength—Guts—Wisdom—Unconditional Love—The ability to STAND TALL

That was the connection between mother and child.

There were more transitions to come as they stepped forward together as mother and daughter. So much had been broken between them for so long, and now they both came to a point where they needed connections.

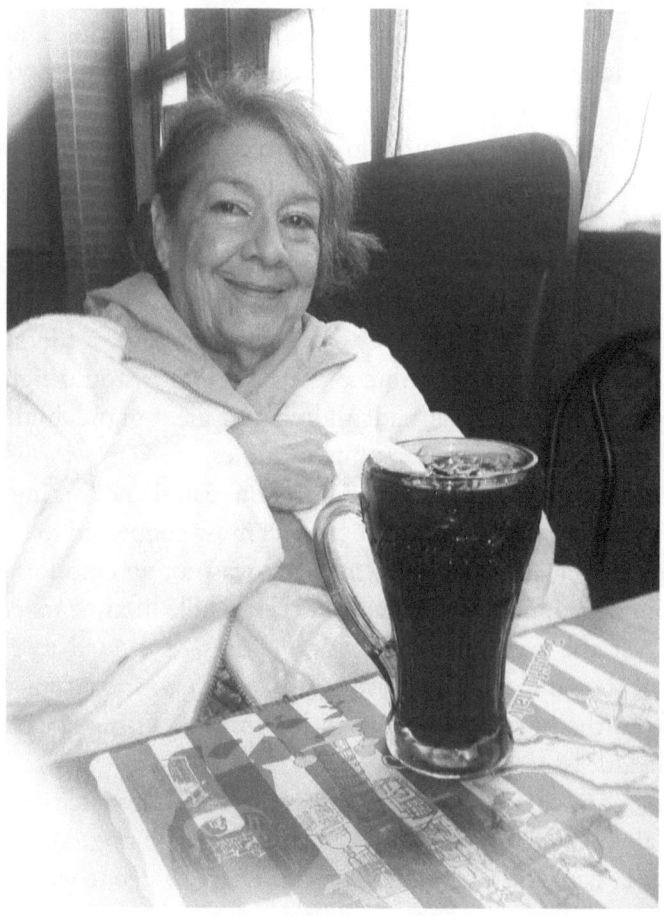

*Lunch*

The conversations became real and heartfelt. This didn't happen all the time because of course mental illness does not let go of the noose for too long, but in between the raindrops, there were more honest conversations.

Joann still had her feisty spirit, and they continued to ride that roller-coaster together as mother and daughter, but there were some good times in between the madness. Lisa loved coming to sit outside with Lil who was another resident at the nursing home. They always chatted, and Lil was a powerhouse with such spunk and spirit. She shared her life stories and both Joann and Lisa listened. It seemed to help them because when Lil shared, it took the pressure off of both of them during times of struggle.

Lisa would bring her children down to visit at times, and even her granddaughter. YES, Joann became a great-grandmother and that made her so very happy. Phoebe would make her laugh and when they visited, they would do art projects together, have pizza and ice cream, and enjoy the time.

The holidays were always the hardest, but Lisa would always try to make it happy for Joann. Christmas was her favorite holiday always, so Lisa would gather her family, cook a full meal, and bring it all down to her mother. She would always reserve a room so they could have privacy and embrace the day. Joann would light up as she spent time with her grandchildren and great-grandchildren. She loved John, and they were smoking buddies.

Many times, Lisa would just stand there in silence taking it all in. It was those moments that made her feel most connected to her mom, because she felt Joann's happiness. That was not an emotion that she felt from her mother very often over their whole lifetime together.

Over the next couple of years, things continued to carry on much of the same way. There were ups and downs, continued phone calls from the nursing home when Joann was causing a ruckus, and more health issues.

Lisa and Joann battled each event as it presented itself. Lisa could also tell Joann's cognitive health was changing, and that was even more concerning to her. When you have someone who struggles with mental illness, and you add in memory loss, this can present a whole new set of issues on a larger scale.

There were more meetings with doctors and staff, and of course, Joann battled every step of the way. She did not make it easy for anyone, especially her daughter, but they continued to move forward.

Lisa kept the visits as regular as possible, bringing along family members as often as she could. Her children were getting older now, with busy lives including work, college, and military duties. Joann was fiercely proud of her grandchildren and bragged about them all of the time. When they did come for visits, she was so excited! It was also nice that they got to see a glimpse of who their grandmother truly was. They did make those important connections with her.

Phoebe, being her first great-grandchild, was the apple of her eye, and she talked about her non-stop. They had so much fun when she came to visit, but as Joann progressed in her physical illnesses, her attitude changed a bit. On the last visit Joann had with Phoebe, Lisa noticed that her mother was very short with her and was even making mean and snarling faces at her.

Lisa addressed her mother, and Joann just lashed out at her in a very negative way. It was at that moment that Lisa realized they were about to come into uncharted waters.

Lisa made the difficult decision not to bring Phoebe down to visit her anymore, as she wanted her memories of "Mo" as she called her to remain positive. Joann stopped talking about her as much as she used to, and that was another sign that things were just not right.

There were more meetings with doctors, and things began to go down-hill from there. Joann was struggling on so many levels, and now she had acute pain in her abdomen. She adamantly refused all testing!

"Nobody is going to fucking touch me! You hear me, Lisa. Do not let them touch me!"

Lisa heard her loud and clear. Joann had enough doctors and testing throughout her life, and she just wanted to be left alone to live out her days as she wanted to.

Lisa clearly understood this, and as her conservator, she called a meeting, stated her mother's wishes, and stood firm against the doctors and nurses that did not agree with her. It was a long-drawn-out meeting, but at the end of the day, Joann got her wishes. No tests!

We were all in agreement that we would call in hospice to help her and keep her comfortable for as long as she needed it. Now that Lisa won that battle for Joann, she had to address Joann's siblings. This was a daunting task in itself, and there were many heated conversations, but again Lisa stood firm wanting to carry out Joann's wishes the best that she could.

Lisa stated over and over again, "I am doing what is best for my mother, and this is her wish, not mine. As her conservator I am in charge. Please respect her wishes."

This was not an easy pill for her family members to swallow, but they didn't have a choice, Lisa was not backing down. Lisa also understood that the family dynamics were very damaged by all of the "unspoken" issues of the past. The dysfunctional upbringing, and the countless traumas along the way. This all added fuel to the fire, but at the end of the day, it was Joann's show!

The one thing about Joann, she was going to direct everything in the way that she wanted it to go. She was a mastermind at making things happen.

As the dust began to settle, family did come to visit her, and now Christmas was upon them. Lisa once again brought down her family, and Joann got to spend her most favorite holiday with her three grandchildren, and now, two great-grandchildren. The room was decorated with snowflakes that Joann and the hospice nurse made together, and the food was endless. There was much chatter going on as she wanted to take in every single moment.

Lisa sat next to her mom to take in all in herself because she knew this very well may be her last Christmas with Joann. It was a mixed bag of emotions because she felt happy seeing her mom happy, but knew the road ahead from here was going to be extremely difficult. Lisa could see that her mother was in a lot of physical pain that day, and she didn't eat very much, which was unlike her. Lisa made all of her favorite dishes, which included lasagna, meatballs, and pumpkin pie. When the day was over and everyone hugged and kissed her goodbye, John and the kids brought everything to the cars, and Lisa wheeled her mom upstairs.

They had a brief conversation about her discomfort, and the nurse came in to give her morphine. As she settled in, she grabbed Lisa's hand.

"Lisa, thank you so much for today. It was incredible to see everyone. I love my little family so much. I love you."

Lisa hugged and kissed her mom's forehead and said, "I love you too mom, very much. I am happy you had a great day. We all did." With that she turned around and left. Joann was already falling off to sleep.

Lisa made her way slowly down that hallway as a few tears

dripped from her eyes. Lisa was deep in thought when she heard a voice, "Hey girl, you."

Lisa turned around, and there was an elderly gentleman sitting in a wheel chair. Lisa had never seen him before in all that time that she had been visiting there. Lisa was also taken aback because this man looked just like her father, who had passed away three years earlier.

"I am Anthony, but everyone calls me Tony," he said. "You must be Joann's daughter. Make sure you drive safely home."

Lisa stared at him in disbelief because the resemblance was uncanny. Lisa finally spoke up and said, "Hi Anthony. I am Joann's daughter. How did you know?"

"You're a West Haven girl who loves the beach. Oh, Savin Rock was a fun place. I know you!"

Lisa did not know how to respond to that, and just said, "Yes we are from West Haven, are you?"

To which he responded, "You could say that."

"Merry Christmas, Anthony. I am sure I will be seeing you around," Lisa said.

"Oh yes you will. I am watching over your mother. She is not feeling well," Anthony replied.

Lisa nodded her head and simply said, "Thank you so much."

She then made her way to the elevator. As she began to step in, she took a glance back at this mysterious man, and he waved to her. Lisa had chills go through her whole body as all she could see was her father. There was a picture that she had of her dad waving, and it was identical. Lisa smiled and boarded the elevator.

All of a sudden, a feeling of comfort washed over her, and she felt as if her mom had a special guardian angel watching over her as she was transitioning from life to death. Again, a huge bag of mixed emotions.

The ride home that night was met with many flashbacks of the past, and a lot of hard things to think about. The face of this mysterious man continued to pop into her head over and over again. After they were home and the kids were all settled in, Lisa shared her experience with her husband who listened intently.

John looked at her and said, "That is your dad, no doubt about it."

Lisa agreed.

Over the next month, Lisa began making several trips to Connecticut because Joann's health was declining rapidly. She encouraged everyone to come visit because she knew that time was precious and the end was closing in on her mother.

Every time Lisa made her way down that hall to her mother's room, Anthony was not far from there. He would always make conversation with Lisa, and the things that he would say would blow her away.

He made many comments and phrases that her father used to do. One day when Lisa was leaving, he called out, "Hey girlie, (he always called me that), enjoy your time at the beach, and be careful going home. You have a long trip back."

Lisa looked him in the eye and said, "How did you know I was going to the beach?"

*It was January in New England, who goes to the beach?*

He responded, "Remember I know you, and that is where you go to think."

Every hair on Lisa's body stood up on end and tingled, and she felt a hot flash come over her.

"Ok, Ok you got me. I am going to the beach, and I promise I will be careful. Take care of my mom until I return, please."

"Of course, you know I will. I have your back," replied Anthony.

"I know you do, thank you," Lisa responded.

Then Anthony reached out his hand, and Lisa took it. He looked at her so intense and seriously as he squeezed her hand tight.

"Remember you were always loved, and that will never go away."

He then smiled at her, and Lisa began to tear up.

"No water works girlie, not today. Go enjoy that beach. I am not going anywhere." Anthony let go of her hand and said, "Go on now."

Lisa blew him a kiss and walked away.

Lisa made her way to the beach in West Haven. The air was crip and cold as it hit her face. There were small snow patches on the sand, and the smell of salt in the air was nurturing. As Lisa walked, she was trying to process everything that was happening, and her meeting with this mysterious man, whom now she believed was her dad in spirit. A mind-blowing revelation!

Lisa always came to the beach in times of trouble. This is

something she had done since she was a young teen.

*How did he know?*

The words that he said were her father's words. Lisa played every conversation over and over in her mind, as it all became very clear to her.

Joann had a guardian angel, and that was her dad. He knew how hard it was going to be for both of them, and he made a divine intervention.

Lisa always had deep faith and love of spirit. Deep within her soul, she knew one hundred percent that Anthony was sent there for a reason, and her dad was the ringleader.

As time moved forward quickly from that day forward, Lisa took great comfort in knowing that her mother was never alone throughout this process of transitioning to the other side. Every time Lisa had a visit with Joann, she also had an insightful conversation with Anthony. The connection was real!

John also met Anthony, and he believed as well. This was truly a divine intervention beyond anyone's control, but spirit.

*Was Joann really coming to the end of her life path?*

*After all the years of pain and struggle, will she find her peace and hold her son in her arms.*

This was something she prayed for every day of her life, since he left this earth. She always talked about the day that she would be reunited with him.

The time was drawing near . . .

*\*\*\*Not all may believe in spirit and divine interventions—that is OK we all have our beliefs. This one happens to be mine, and I am honored to have a glimpse into the unknown. Lisa Zarcone*

# Chapter 23

# The Time Is Now

Throughout the last few months of Joann's life, she showed such great courage, and strength. She never lost her faith in God, or hope that things would be OK. She always ran the show, and it was her show; large, grand, and chaotic just like her personality! Joann gallantly made her way to the end of her life path, with her daughter Lisa by her side as always. Joann knew deep down inside that Lisa would never falter. She depended on her right to the very end.

Lisa continued to support her decisions, with much badgering from her family, but she knew what was best for her mother—and that was to let her die with dignity. These were her wishes, not her daughter's, so Lisa stood by her side and made sure all of her demands were granted.

Our mysterious man, "Anthony," was always in the background. It was like he was waiting in the wings of a massive Broadway play. Lisa would see him in the doorway of her mother's room every single time she was there. He would always give a smile and a wave.

Family and friends continued to come for visits to say goodbye to Joann. At times, it seemed like a never-ending flow of people! Some people she hadn't seen in years. It amazed Lisa that they waited until the end to finally show up! This alone caused her to feel a mixed bag of emotions. The pings and twinges of the past bellowing in her ear.

Joann had a really hard time in the last few days of her life. It was so very hard to watch her suffer once again, as she had been through so much in her life. We all prayed for her to go peacefully, and Lisa sat with her playing music, and talking to her about the good times that they shared together.

In a brief moment of clarity Joann opened her eyes and looked directly at her daughter.

"Lisa, I am so sorry for what I put you through. You know how much I love you. When I am gone, can I please come back and visit you?"

Lisa held her hand tight and said to her, "Mom, I love you more than anything, and of course you can. I will be happily waiting for your signs."

Joann closed her eyes resting for a bit as the exhaustion from speaking washed over her face, and then, all of a sudden, she had a little burst of energy, and she started singing:

"*Bye, Bye, Miss American Pie . . . this will be the day that I die . . .*"

It was eerie, but Lisa knew in her heart and soul that it was Joann's way of telling her that her time here on this earth was just about over.

Joann always had a great fear that she would die alone, or her daughter would be alone with her when she died. She always said that when she passed away, the only two people that she wanted there was her sister and daughter. She was very adamant about her wishes, and she talked about this many, many times as it came closer to the end. It was like she willed it to be. On the day of her death that was far from the case. Her fears were clearly put to rest because she was surrounded by many people.

The nurses and doctors, along with hospice were so very kind and loving to her. They embraced Joann for who she was, and why she did the things that she would do. It was there that she found acceptance, respect, and peace.

Lisa came in that morning, and Joann was sleeping. She was not talking anymore. Lisa was sitting with her mom in deep thought when her aunt randomly showed up. She was quite surprised to see her standing there. She stated that she had a really funny feeling, and she heard her sister say *come now*, so she felt compelled to do so. Lisa shared with her aunt that the same thing happened to her as well.

They hung out for a while making small talk, and then the hospice nurse encouraged them to go get some coffee and stretch their legs for a bit. She assured them that Joann was not going anywhere just yet, and her vital signs were still very strong. So, they listened to the nurse and reluctantly decided to go for that walk, making their way down to the cafeteria.

As they sat for a few moments talking, Lisa had a funny feeling come rushing over her, and she felt the chills and tingling throughout her whole body. She instantly looked at the clock: it was 1:10 p.m. She abruptly said, "Let's go back upstairs. I really feel like something is happening this very moment."

Lisa and her aunt made their way back upstairs, as her aunt was looking at her with a very concerned look. They made their way down the long hallway and back into Joann's room. Lisa instantly could tell she was dying.

Lisa's face started burning as she went over to her to take her hand and said, "Mom it is ok to go. I love you so very much."

She then placed her hand on her mother's chest, and Joann gave her one final gift of love before leaving this earth, and it was feeling her last heartbeat. Lisa was in awe of the feeling as she embraced it so deeply. She could feel the energy travel right up her arm, and then, just like that, there was nothing. There was instant silence.

Lisa looked at her aunt and said, "I think she is gone!"

She told her to go get the nurse, and her aunt went barreling down the hallway to the nurse's station. They all came running down the hall like a football team running onto the field. As Lisa watched them rush into the room, she already knew she was gone, as she felt her leave. She also saw a flash of light, and a glimpse of her dad and brother, as she turned to leave the room.

The nurse confirmed she was gone, and my aunt turned to me.

"Just like that! That's it!"

I said, "YES!"

We all just stood there for a moment taking it all in. There was a moment of silence, and then one of the nurses began to sing. She was of Jamaican culture, and she sang the most beautiful song in her native language. As we stood there listening to this beautiful melody, Lisa scanned the room, watching the doctors and nurses holding hands and crying. Joann touched many lives right until the end.

When the song ended, the staff slowly left the room, offering their condolences to Lisa and her aunt. Lisa thought for a few moments, and said out loud to her aunt, "It is over. All the years of her pain and suffering are now over.

All the years of her abuse that she bestowed upon us, and so many others, are over just like that, peaceful and calm."

Her aunt nodded her head in silence, as she just sat there taking it all in. It seemed as if she was making peace with her sister. Her silent thoughts and feelings she sent out to Joann. It was for her ears only!

After a little bit of time, Lisa told her aunt it was ok to leave, and she would take care of all the arrangements. They hugged, and Lisa walked over to the door with her.

There was Anthony sitting in his wheel chair right outside the door. Lisa had caught a glimpse of him in the doorway earlier when her mother was transitioning.

He looked at Lisa and her aunt.

"I am very sorry for your loss. She was a good-hearted woman."

They thanked him, and Lisa's aunt walked away. As Lisa was watching her walk down the hallway, she turned back around to speak with Anthony, but he was gone. Lisa was a bit puzzled, as he was just there in his wheelchair.

Lisa walked back in the room feeling a bit confused and thinking about the whole experience that just transpired in front of her eyes. The only term Lisa could think of was "Mind Blowing" as she stood there taking in the moment.

The years upon years of her mother's mania was over in just one breath. She was finally at peace, and that gave Lisa comfort. Lisa also knew that Anthony was instrumental in helping guide her mother home, and for that she would be forever grateful.

**Lisa's Thoughts & Feelings about her experience . . .**

At 1:17 p.m. my mother left this earth, with my father and brother by her side guiding her home, as she wanted. She spoke of them being there a few times in those last days, but she told them she was not ready, they needed to come back. This was so her: she waited forty-three years to hug my brother, but she told him to wait.

*Why?*

I know that answer: she did not want me to be alone at the moment of her passing. She wanted her sister there with me, and she orchestrated it. When I had the feeling, something was wrong, it was 1:10 (this is my father's birthday) and the moment of her last breath 1:17 (March 17th, my brother's birthday). It all made perfect sense to me. It all had meaning as she wanted it to be. Nobody else but her!

She always said, "I Choose Life." But when she could not choose life anymore, she chose to die on her terms, with strength, pride, and dignity. My mother did it HER way right until the end. There could be no other way. She demanded her final moment be about HER.

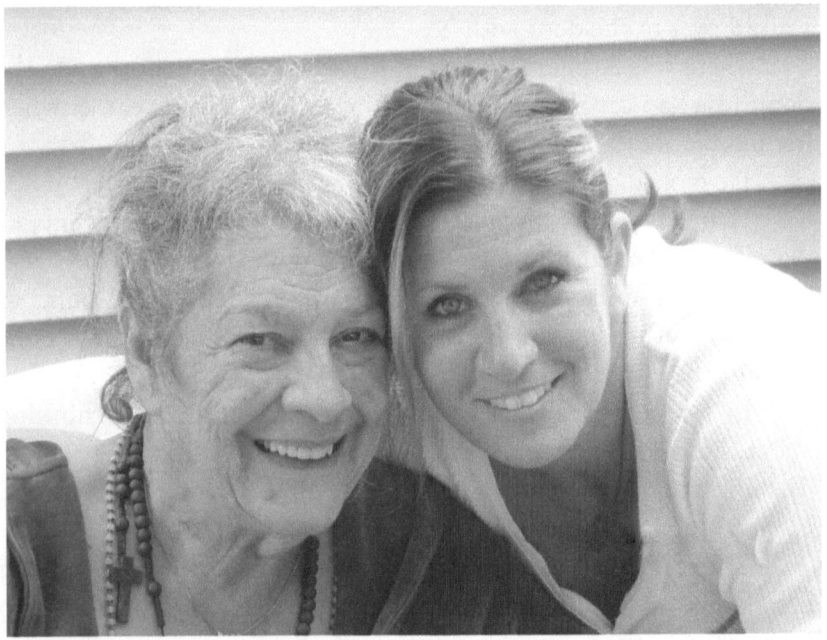

*Mom's Birthday 2011*

I love my mother with all my heart, and I miss her every single day. Honestly, I do not miss her mania, but I do miss her the true Joann Sega. I am extremely proud to call her my mother. I learned many valuable lessons from her, and I have many of her beautiful qualities.

My mother did tell me over and over constantly, throughout the years,

"Lisa, you must write a book about me and one about our life together. You will make millions!"

She also told me that our family was very special and unique.

"Lisa, there will never be another story like this one ever! It must be told to help others who continue to struggle. We need to bring awareness to mental illness." Joann's words!

I feel she had the wisdom to know the truth about many things. I believe she is correct. Our story is quite unique and different. My mother knew many things way beyond the realms of this world, and she saw things in a very unique light. I do believe she gave me that incredible gift as well.

As my mother's life has now come to a close, it is certainly not the end. Her light, love, and spirit lives on inside of me, and all who truly loved her. Her legacy is being honored as we (her family) step forward, knowing how much she loved us all. She taught us all the true meaning of family loyalty. Joann was loyal to her family even through the illness and mania. Her heart always remained true.

Writing this book, *The Book of Joann*, was a true honor and privilege. I heard her voice many times whispering in my ear, because I know she was conducting this whole journey, that is now complete.

So, there it is.

Now you know the true story of this incredible, strong-willed, beautiful woman—

The story of Joann Helen Sabatasso Sega a true Life Warrior.

Always loved and never to be forgotten!

Love you always mom, as you now walk with the angels.

LIGHT
LOVE
PEACE

# Chapter 24

# Epilogue—"24"

As I have said countless times, Joann always ran the show. It is fitting that the Epilogue would be Chapter 24, as this is her birthday:
June 24th.

Writing my mother's story was truly challenging for me, for so many reasons. First of all, going back to the beginning of her life before I even existed was an experience in itself. I had to tap into my memories, and my mother's writings to put it all together. Joann always shared her countless stories, and I was her loyal student, taking in every single word. I had a deep curiosity about this mysterious woman that I called "Mom."

As I wrote this book, I could clearly hear my mother speaking to me as the story came together. I had many powerful moments on this writing journey. I learned new things about Joann and gained a new respect for her, as I was now seeing life through her eyes. I wrote this story from her perspective. I have to be honest in saying, this was one of the hardest things I have ever accomplished in my adult life.

As I made my way forward into the chapters about our life together, I had to keep an open mind and heart to continue to see it from her point of view. Did I have pings of pain bellowing in from the past, ABSOLUTELY!

I was also given the opportunity to heal on new levels. Having to relive those horrendous moments were quite painful, but I found clarity and healing through the many emotions and tears.

*The Book of Joann* offered me another chance at healing my mind, body and spirit. I am grateful for this journey.

Am I healed fully?

I have to say that I do not believe people can fully heal one hundred percent, because the damage has been done. What I can say is that I feel as close to fully healing as one could be. There will always be pings of the past that pop up once and a while. I have learned how to let them in, embrace them, and return them to the universe.

My dad told me a long time ago, "Always Move Forward."

I believe that is the best advice anyone can offer someone who has dealt with pain and trauma. Keep on moving as you lay the past to rest. You can look back for a moment, give it a wink, but do not get stuck there.

*What does the future hold from here as this book is finally published?*

My goal for my mother's story is to bring further awareness to Mental Illness and all of the stigmas that are still attached to it. By sharing my mother's powerful story, I hope that this gives other people who are struggling silently the strength and courage to step into the light and break that darkness once and for all.

I will use my story, *The Unspoken Truth, A Memoir* and *The Book Of Joann*, as learning tools of how it all falls apart if people who are struggling are not supported properly.

My mother did not get the proper help and support that she needed, and because of that, we both fell through the cracks of a flawed system.

My story is hideous. NO child should ever have to endure what I did, but the harsh reality is that far too many children are living my past nightmare right now!

I hope that by sharing my mother's story, I can change that reality. The more that we talk about these hard subjects that need to be addressed, we are pushing for change. We are pushing to be heard, and we will never be silenced again.

So, there it is as promised. I have shared two very powerful stories for purpose. I always knew that I would do this, as I believe it was my destiny.

I step forward with courage, strength, and deep faith.

My voice is strong, and I will always advocate for the voiceless.

The time is now for change, and I am going to be the playmaker on this next leg of the journey.

Thank you Joann for raising an incredibly strong daughter. I walk with my head held high, love in my heart, and a fierce passion for change.

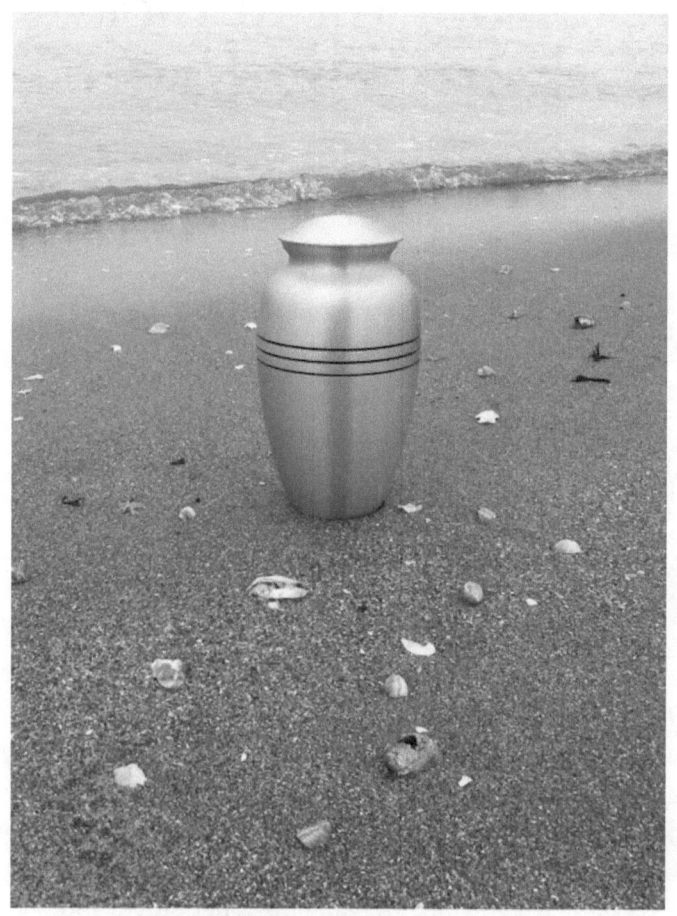

*I promised mom I would take her to the ocean.*

God Bless & Embrace The Journey
Lisa Rose Sega Zarcone
Life Warrior—Survivor

# About the Author

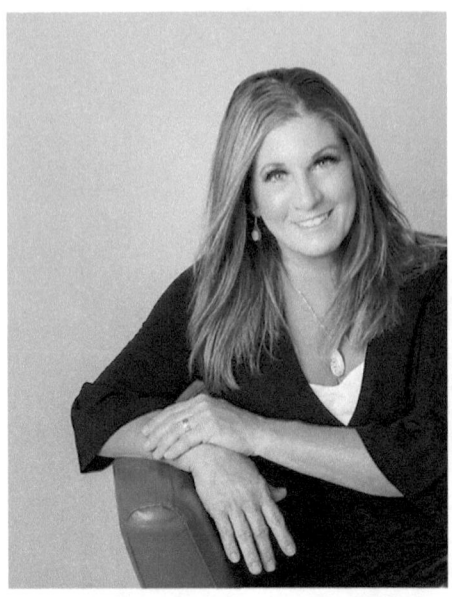

**Lisa Zarcone** is one remarkable woman. Her childhood was nothing less than hideous. Her ability to survive in her silent world of treachery is truly astonishing. A wife, mother of three, and grandmother of three (Memah), Lisa is the everyday woman with an extraordinary gift for giving and is full of passion.

Lisa gained her voice by validating her story, and she healed through the process. She was able to see the view and perspective of the people in her life, and that is where she found forgiveness. Lisa has a passion for working with those who have mental illness. What her past has taught her about mental illness cannot be read in a textbook.

"I am a voice for the voiceless, and through my voice, I hope to promote healing."

Lisa's motto is "Embrace The Journey" because you never know what life will hand you next.

Lisa is currently the Massachusetts National Ambassador for NAASCA (National Association of Adult Survivors of Child Abuse). She is spreading awareness for child safety/abuse and mental health illness/stigmas. She travels all over to publicly speak as she is working towards raising awareness, educating people, and promoting change in a very flawed system as too many children continue to fall through the cracks. She continues to work effortlessly as this is her passion, mission, and goal to break the silence.

Lisa was honored in the "2023 Women of Impact" by *Business West Magazine* (Western Massachusetts).

She has worked with disabled children and adults teaching life skills and writing. She also served as a mentor to young women in a locked-down facility teaching journaling, poetry, and art therapy. She has also done a lot of work advocating for Suicide Prevention and Post Raumatic Stress Disorder (PTSD) Awareness.

Lisa inspires others through her social media platforms, offering encouragement, motivation, kindness, empathy, compassion and inspiration. She is always approachable, and answers every message sent to her.

## Another Book by Lisa Zarcone

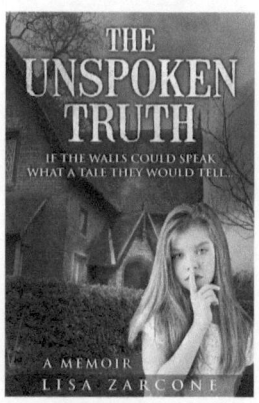

Lisa took all of her past experiences of her personal trauma and abuse and wrote a detailed, personal memoir of her life. She shares her story through the eyes of herself as a child. She gives the reader a first-hand view of abuse through the child's perspective. This is a very raw and real look at her life as it played out. Lisa left her story very choppy, as the clouded mind of an abused child is in continued fight and flight mode trying to survive each day seeing through a clouded lens. It is powerful and devasting at the same time, reading her story.

www.ingramcontent.com/pod-product-compliance
Lightning Source LLC
LaVergne TN
LVHW040050080526
838202LV00045B/3563